Scientific Turkey Farming

Scientific Turkey Farming

Authors :

D. THYAGARAJAN
A. ASHOK

SSPH

SATISH SERIAL PUBLISHING HOUSE
403, Express Tower, Commercial Complex, Azadpur, Delhi-110033 (India)
Phone : 011-27672852, Fax : 91-11-27672046
E-mail :info@satishserial.com, hkjain1975@yahoo.com
Website : www.satishserial.com

Published by :

SATISH SERIAL PUBLISHING HOUSE
403, Express Tower, Commercial Complex, Azadpur, Delhi-110033 (INDIA)
Phone : 011-27672852 Fax : 91-11-27672046
E-mail : info@satishserial.com, hkjain1975@yahoo.com

ISBN 978-93-81226-18-6

Typeset at: Harminder Singh Kharb *for* Laxmi Art Creation
Printed at: Salasar Imaging Systems, Delhi-110035

PREFACE

Scientific turkey farming comprises of forty chapters on different aspects of scientific turkey farming , feeds and feeding and hatchery management. In this book all technological interventions and scientific know how to on scientific rearing and housing, poult management, grower management, layer management, breeder management are discussed. Feeding management for turkeys at different age group based on seasonal management is also discussed in detail. It covers turkeys flock health and biosecurity. Product technology aspects such as nutritive value of egg and meat and its processing and a way how to market the product is elaborated. As to encourage the entrepreneurs, information regarding bank loan and insurance, bank norms and interest rates are given. As to keep the profitable farm, record keeping and types of records to be maintained with a model format is discussed. Manufacturing of compound feed and technique involved are discussed. The feeding management is very quite important in turkey farming. All about, feed, feeding of brooder, grower, layer and breeder along with nutrient requirement are presented. Computation of ration and preparation ration for different age groups of turkey are also outlined. Establishment of feed mill and feed milling process is also discussed. In hatchery management, formation and structure of egg, embryonic development, factors required for incubation, hatchery designs, hatchery hygiene and hatching ability of turkey egg are narrated in detail.

Being the first book of turkey farming, it will give definitely over all idea to new entrepreneur, scientific outline for students on identified new technological intervention for sustainable turkey farming.

Authors

CONTENTS

□□□

Chapter 1

Turkey Farming - Present Status

In India, sixty percent of the population is dependant on agriculture and allied activities. However the contribution of this sector to the gross domestic product is less than 20%. Although India is self sufficient in food production, it is yet to attain nutritional security. This can be overcome by augmenting the production of protein rich animal products like milk, egg and meat. Livestock and poultry farming are potential income generating activities in rural areas which can improve the economic status of the rural poor.

Among poultry, turkey occupies an important position next to chicken in the world. They are reared only for meat and its meat is the leanest among poultry.

Turkey Farming in India

In India, turkey is reared mainly for meat. It is growing in stature as an important poultry enterprise. They are capable of growing in any agro climatic conditions. It is reared mostly in rural areas in backyard. Scientific practices are yet to be adopted in a large scale. In urban areas consumption of turkey meat is gaining popularity. Kerala and Tamil Nadu are the leading states in turkey production. Non-descriptive turkeys are found in good numbers in Kerala, Tamil Nadu, eastern districts of Uttar Pradesh and other parts of India. The three commonly found varieties of turkey in India are Broad Breasted Bronze, Broad Breasted White and Beltsville Small White. Presently, elite turkey stocks are maintained in Tamilnadu Veterinary and Animal Sciences University, Chennai; Central Avian Research Institute, Barielly; Central Poultry Development organization, Hesserghatta and other state government farms.

Turkeys are no longer seasonal "crop". It is being produced round the year and all sections of the society consume it without any taboo. They can be reared with a minimum investment. They are marketed between 16 to 24 weeks of age depending upon the requirement and market condition. Turkey farming is a prospective micro entrepreneurial avenue and can definitely improve the economic status of small and marginal farmers. Farmers who have been not able to hold on to the changing trends in broiler and layer industry are also switching on to turkey rearing as an alternate farming. Therefore it is necessary to promote turkey farming in a large way.

Turkeys can easily be started by hatching eggs or by raising young poults. They can be grown and home processed without the use of expensive processing equipment, or they may be sold to live markets.

Advantages of Turkey Farming

- Turkey meat is considered a delicacy.
- The meat is tender, tastier and contains less fat than chicken.
- They are more disease resistant than hybrid chicken.
- They are more ideally suited for semi intensive or range system of rearing.
- Number of vaccinations are fewer.
- Meat is always sold at a premium price.
- Egg is nutritious and contains quality protein.
- Turkeys are good foragers - the feed cost can be minimized.

Disadvantages of Turkey Farming

- Critical inputs like day old turkey poults, hatching eggs, and turkey feed are not easily available.
- Management of turkey poults are more difficult than chicks.
- Tom turkeys are heavy in size. So they are not able to mate the hens frequently and hence the fertility rate is low in turkeys.
- Feed conversion efficiency of turkeys is much lesser than chicken (8-24 weeks).
- Heavier body weight of turkeys, restrict the retail sales of turkey meat to a large extent.

Chapter 2

Varieties of Turkey

Turkeys are native to North America. They belong to the order Galliformes, along with Chickens. There are two species of wild Turkey: the North American Wild Turkey (*Meleagris gallopavo*) and the Central American Ocellated Turkey (*M. ocellata*). The modern domesticated turkey was developed from the North American Wild Turkey by the indigenous people of Mexico (Aztecs). Turkeys were taken to Europe by the Spanish, who found them as a favourite domesticated animal among the Aztecs. The Aztecs used turkeys as a source of protein (meat and eggs) and the feathers for decoration.

The "breeds" of turkeys often referred to are actually varieties that originated from the North American wild turkey. The seven standard varieties recognized by the American Poultry association are Bronze, White Holland, Bourbon Red, Narragansett, Black, Slate and Beltsville Small White. The two varieties that are not recognized are Broad-Breasted Bronze, Broad-Breasted White. (also called Large White).The most commonly raised commercial variety is the Large

White. The Broad-Breasted Bronze, similar in size and conformation, is less popular because of a preference for white feathering.

The major primary breeders of turkeys in the world are:

- British United Turkeys
- Hybrid Turkeys
- Nicholas Turkey

They offer 10 parental strains Big 6, Big-9, BUT-8, BUT-9, BUT-10, Hybrid converter, Hybrid Grade maker, Hybrid XL, Nicholas 900 & Nicholas 300.

Broad Breasted Bronze

The plumage colour is black with an iridescent sheen of red, green and bronze. The beak is light horn at tip and dark at base. The colour of the throat wattle is red changeable to bluish white. The beards are black. The shank and toes are dull black in young and smoky pink in mature birds. Of all meat animals, the Broad Breasted Bronze uniformly produces well fleshed carcass.

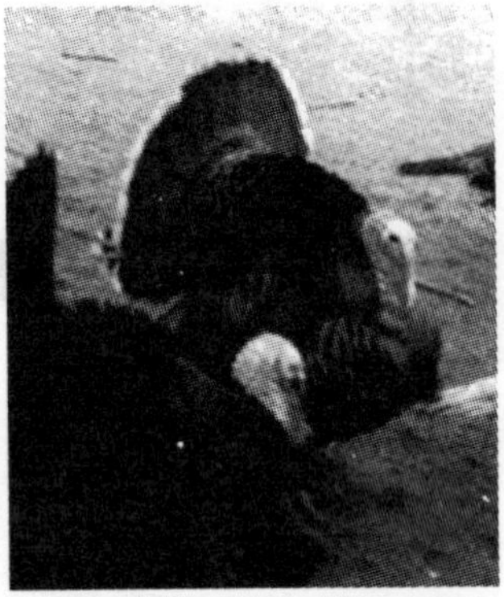

Broad Breasted Bronze

Body Weight

Male : 16 kg

Female : 9 kg

Broad Breasted White

This was developed in 1950 in Cornell University of America. This is a hybrid of Broad Breasted Bronze and White Holland. The plumage is solid white in colour. The beak is light pinkish horn. The colour of throat wattle is red changeable to pinkish white. The fertility rate of this variety is higher than both the parents. Commercial rearing of turkey is mainly based on this variety.

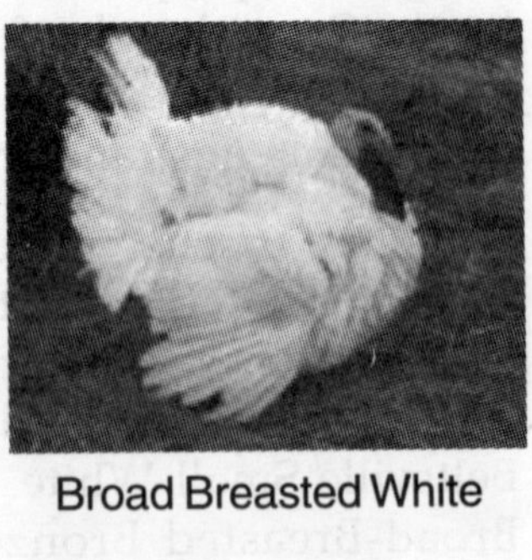

Broad Breasted White

Body Weight

Male : 15 kg

Female : 8 kg

Beltsville Small White

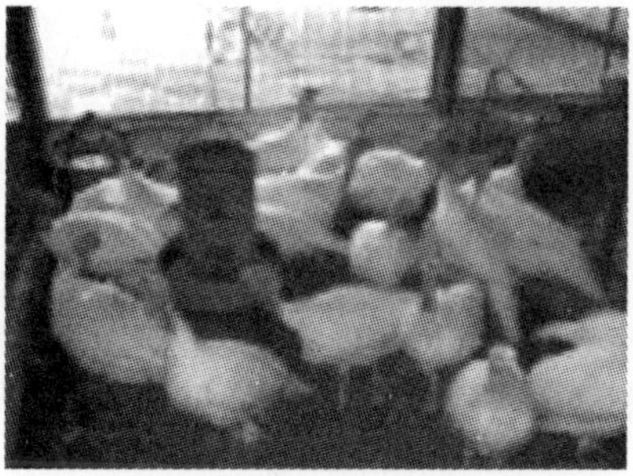

Beltsville small white

This was developed in United States Agricultural Research Institute. This variety was popularized all over the world from 1941 to 1962. This resembles Broad Breasted White variety in its colour and external appearance but, is smaller in size. The egg production rate, fertility, and hatching ability are higher in this variety than the others; but the brooding ability of this variety is lower when compared to others.

Body Weight

Male : 8 kg

Female : 4 kg

White Holland

This variety of turkey was developed from Bronze variety. The plumage of this variety appears solid white in colour.

Body Weight

Male : 15 kg

Female : 8 kg

Narragansett

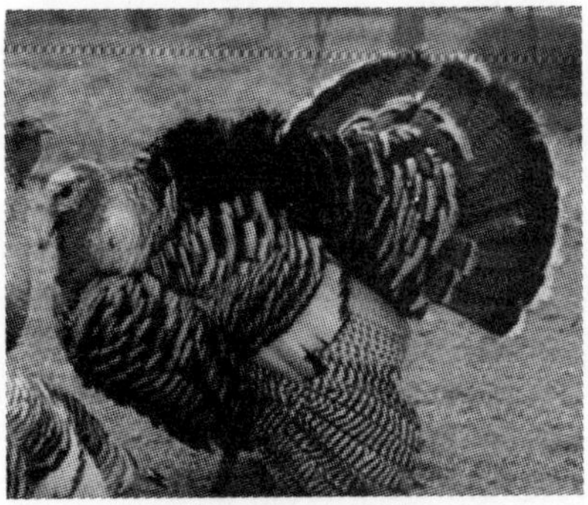

Narragansett

This variety was developed in Rhode island of America by crossing between country and wild turkeys. The plumage of this variety is grayish black in colour with white markings. The colour of throat wattle is red changeable to bluish white. The beard is black. In adults the shank and toes are deep salmon.

Body Weight

Male : 15 kg
Female : 8 kg

Bourbon Red

This variety was developed in Kentucky, America. The plumage is brownish red with white wing and tail markings. The beak is light horn at tip and dark at base. The colour of throat wattle is red changeable to bluish white. The shank and toes are reddish pink in adults.

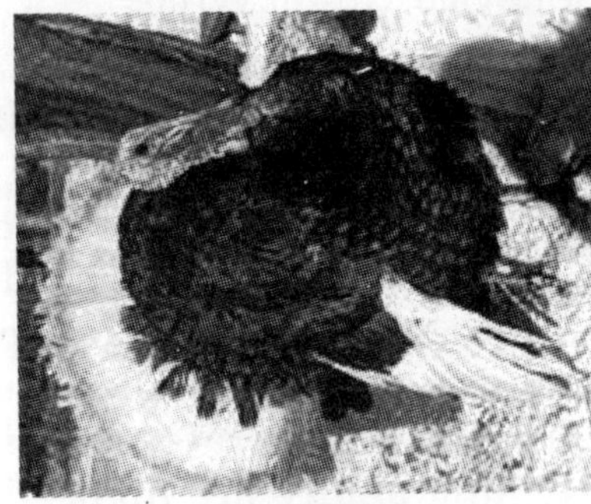
Bourbon Red

Body Weight

Male : 15 kg
Female : 8 kg

Black

This variety of turkey is reared in Spain, Italy, and France. The plumage colour is metallic black. The beak is slate black. The colour of throat wattle is red changeable to bluish white. The beard is black. The shank and toes are pink in adults.

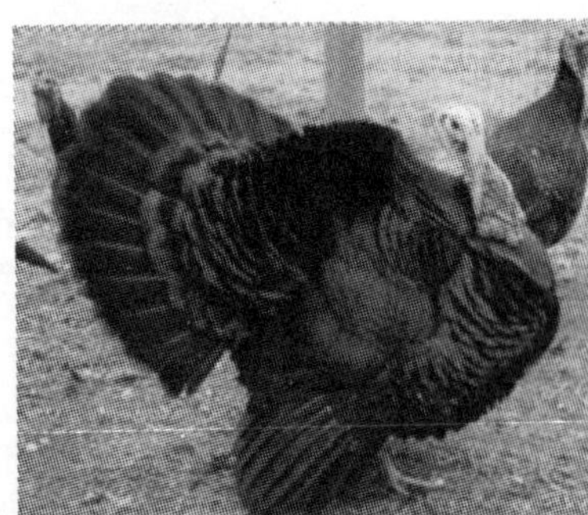
Black

Body Weight

Male : 15 kg
Female : 8 kg

Economic traits (Beltsville Small White Variety)

Male : female sex ratio	1:3 or 1:4
Average egg weight	75 g
Average weight of day old turkey poult	50 g
Age at sexual maturity	24 to 28 weeks

contd...

Average egg production/female / year		80 to 100 eggs
Average turkey poults obtained / female/year		50 to 60
Incubation period		28 days
Highest egg production period		28 - 52 weeks
Market age	Male	16 to 24 weeks
	Female	18 to 24 weeks
Market weight 24 weeks	Male	4.0 to 4.5 kg
	Female	3.0 to 3.5 kg
Feed intake till market	Male	16 to 18 kg
24 weeks	Female	12 to 14 kg
Feed conversion ratio (24 weeks)		4.0 to 4.5 kg
Mortaility rate during first 8 weeks		3% to 4%

❐❐❐

Chapter 3

Systems of Rearing and Housing

Systems of Rearing

Basically there are three systems of rearing the birds. System of rearing will depend on the amount of money that can be invested, place of rearing, number of birds, etc. The three types are as follows:

1. Free Range System

In this system of management, the birds are free to move about in an open area. (Unrestricted movement) The birds have more time to access the open area. Shelters or natural shades are recommended for range production. If shelters are provided they must in adequate numbers/space to prevent over crowding.

Disadvantages

- Management problems encountered, especially during disease outbreaks.

- Large area is required to rear the birds.
- High proportion of dirty eggs.

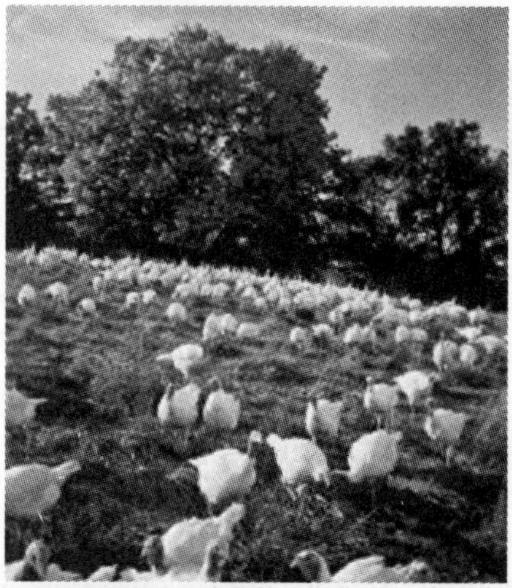

Free range system

2. Semi Range System

This system most often uses an existing farm building usually open fronted with an adjoining yard. This system probably survives mainly for small domestic flocks, where it is more convenient to set aside a small amount of land for their exclusive use than to have them roaming at large.

Advantages

- This system avoids the need to shut up birds at night.
- Capital costs low.
- Hens have continuous daytime access to open air runs.

Disadvantages

- Build up of disease.
- High proportion of dirty eggs.

3. Intensive Rearing System

a. Deep Litter

The maximum stocking is not more than seven hens per square meter of floor space.

Advantages

- Easy to manage the flock.
- High proportion of clean egg production.

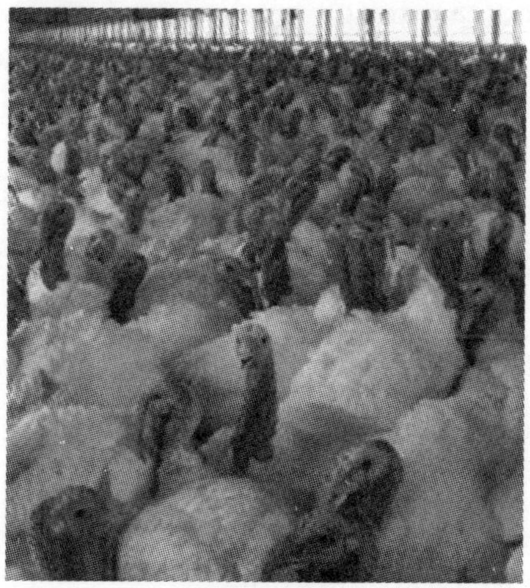

Deep Litter

b. Cage System

Cage rearing system can be adopted in day old turkey poults till they attain 8 weeks of age.

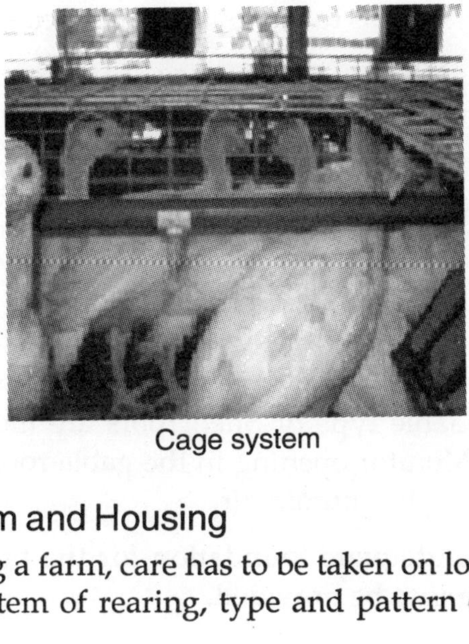

Cage system

Location of Farm and Housing

Before staring a farm, care has to be taken on location of the farm, site selection, system of rearing, type and pattern of the houses, etc.

Poultry need housing mainly to protect them from predator, theft, adverse climatic conditions and management and to provide ideal conditions for optimum performance. An ideal or a well constructed poultry house is one which helps conserve the bird's energy, make for economy in feed, increase in egg production, improve fertility, promote health and growth and keep the mortality at low level.

Site Selection

The following points have to be borne in mind before site selection:

- The farm has to be located away from residential and industrial area.
- A virgin area is most preferred to all other areas.
- The farm is to be located within 50 kms from the marketing area, on the out skirts of the city, village or town.
- The site selected is to be at least 1 km away from other nearby poultry farm to avoid infection.
- The farm is to have good access to market area; the road has to be motorable, for easy transportation of farm input and output.
- A three phase electricity supply is to be always available to the farm.
- The selected land has to be elevated and rectangular to the extent possible.
- More than sufficient potable (drinking) water is to be always available for farm and farm personnel use.
- The selected sight is not to be situated in low lying or water logging area.
- Sufficient space has to be available for future expansion.

Basics of Building Design

- *Roof Type* - Gable type or Shed roofs are most preferred over other roofs. Monitor opening in the gable roof is also helpful to allow escape of hot humid air.
- *Foundation* - Adequate foundation for the building other than pole building is to be provided.

- *Floor* - Concrete floor is highly desirable for cage and floor types for ease in cleaning and for effective disinfection.
- *Walls* - Solid portion of the wall is constructed with durable material impervious to moisture.

Design for Individual Building

Orientation and Spacing

East- West Orientation is preferred. To achieve maximum air movement, houses have to be perpendicular to the prevailing wind direction.

Distance between the Buildings

Spacing between the buildings is of great importance to prevent disease spread and better ventilation (minimum 30 feet).

Building Width

In naturally ventilated houses, the width can not be more than 30 feet. Narrower houses are preferred in hot humid climates.

Building Length

This can be of any convenient length. In long buildings, doors are often required to be constructed in the side walls at the suitable distances for services and bird removal.

Height of the Shed

The height of the farm house depends upon the type of roofing. Normally, in all types of roofing the height of the house has to be about 10 to 12 feet. In cage house the height has to be above 15 feet. The height of the side wall along with the net has to be 6 to 7 feet.

Sidewalls

The height of the sidewall has to be 1.5 feet. Nets/welded mash has to be fitted for a height of 5 feet above the side walls. The width of the side walls has to be 4.5 inches.

Roof Overhang

The roofs need to have an overhang of 3 feet on all sides to prevent rain from blowing inside the house. It is necessary to slope the overhang toward the ground.

Doors

The doors have to open outwards in one direction only.

Lighting Facility

The lights fixed have to be 7 to 8 feet above the floor level. The maximum distance between two 60 watts bulbs has to be 10 feet. The distance between two tubes has to be 15 feet.

Types of Houses

- Brooder house (0 to 8 weeks)
- Grower house (9 to 24 weeks)
- Layer house (above 24 weeks)
- Cage housing of turkey(0 to 8 weeks)

Poultry Farm Equipments

The equipments used in poultry houses have to be simple, easy to use and durable. Their cleaning and disinfections have to be easy. The equipments can be listed as follows:

Brooder Equipment

Brooder equipments are used to provide warmth and light and to rear the poults during the first few weeks of life. The brooders consist of a heating source, reflectors to reflect the heat and light towards the chicks. Depending on the heating source or fuel, different types available are;

- Electrical brooders
- Gas brooders
- Coal/charcoal brooders
- Kerosene wick stove brooders

The electrical brooders use infrared bulbs, incandescent bulbs, heating filaments or coils with thermostat device or special focus bulbs, which reflect the heat downwards. Gas brooders are used wherever gas is cheaper or in farms where "bio-gas" is produced by using cage droppings or cattle dung. Coal, charcoal, wood, lignite and kerosene wick stoves are used as brooders in places where electricity is not available or costly and where power failure is quite common. The centralised heating system is adopted in environmentally controlled poultry houses. Here the entire brooder house is heated to 32°C using electricity, gas, coal, etc. as fuel.

For effective utilization of heat and light generated from the brooders, some other reflecting device, usually made up of polished or enamel coated metal are used, to focus the heat towards the poults. Metal canopy (open umbrella shaped), hover or even metallic lampshades with adjustable stands or hanging devices are used for this purpose.

Chick Guards

Chick guards are thin sheets of metal, hard board, cardboard or bamboo mat of 35 to 45 cm height and of varying lengths. They are used to restrict the movement of chicks, so that the chicks can be kept closer to the brooders and prevent them from chilling. Moreover, it is used to round off the sharp corners, and thereby prevents trampling of chicks during night time, vaccination, debeaking and catching.

Feeders

Feeders are equipments used to feed the birds, by placing feed in them. They may be conventional, semi-automatic or automatic of various designs and shapes such as linear, circular of hanging type, made up of either metal or plastic.

Waterers

Waterers or drinkers are used to provide water to the birds. Like feeders, waterers are available in different sizes, designs and shapes. They may be conventional, semi-automatic or automatic channels, consists of cups, nipples or basins, made up of metal, plastic or both.

Debeakers

Automatic de-beaking equipment is available.

Vaccinators

- Automatic Vaccinator
- Fowl pox Vaccinator
- Needle with syringe

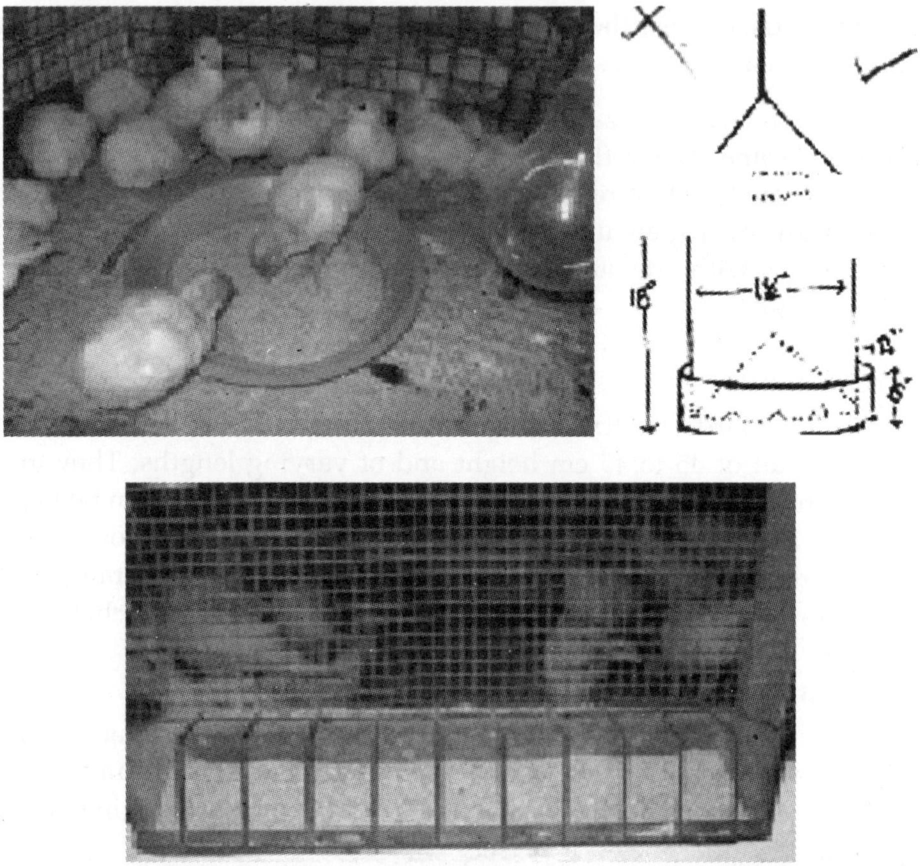

Feeders

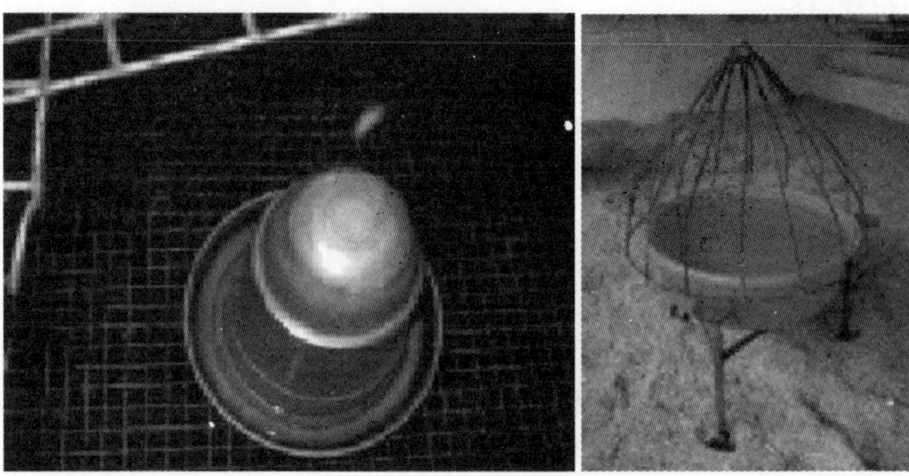

Waterers

Miscellaneous Equipments

- Nest
- Rake
- Shovels
- Egg and chick weighing balance
- Sprayer
- Buckets
- Egg filler flats
- Trolleys
- Incinerator
- Flame gun (or) Blowlamp
- Vacuum Dust Cleaner
- Weighing machines/balance
- Measuring jar or cylinder

□□□

Chapter 4

Poult Management

Great care has to be provided for the management of turkey poults. Turkey poults are capable growing very fast. As a result, upto 8 weeks of age they are fed with high protein diet to enable them grow faster. Feed containing vitamins and anticoccidials are also to be provided. Turkeys are termed as poults from day old to 8 weeks of age; from 9 weeks to 24 weeks they are called as turkey growers; and from 24 weeks when they start laying eggs they are called as turkey layers/ breeders.

Day-old poults, weigh 45-50 grams. They are transported to the turkey farm within 24 hours of hatch. Boxes of live poults are to be handled in a level position and never thrown. Poults are removed by tilting the box slightly and pushing the birds out carefully, or by inclining the box slowly and then withdrawing it from under them with a smooth, swift movement. When removed by hand (with the hands forming a scoop) the poults must not be squeezed. They should be dropped more than 15 cm on a hard floor or 30 cm on a soft floor.

Importance of Brooder House Management

Livability is the keyword as it relates to turkey brooder house management. Percent livability in the brooder house is a good indicator of future flock performance. Economic loss from early poult mortality is not confined to poult cost as greater economic loss often is experienced in the future performance of the surviving poults.

In a brooding and growing program from 0 to 8 weeks old, the following performance is expected.

Hen poults—97% livability

Tom poults—95% livability

Before procuring the poults the following points are to be considered. To compensate the mortality in the turkey poults, 5% extra poults are to be procured at the beginning. Begin with good quality poults. Secure poults from breeders tested negative for Salmonella and *PPLO*.

Poult Quality Assessment

It is important to assess the quality of each hatch received. They may be different due to the following factors:

- Age of breeder flock
- First egg poults
- Breeder nutrition
- Heat stress
- Hatchery profile
- Hatchery sanitation
- Age of egg set
- Egg handling, storage and sanitation

When poults arrive, check a representative sample for the following:

Dehydration can be a major factor in mortality during the first 3 days in the farm.

Signs of Dehydration

- Skin over the legs appears oedemakom.
- Blood vessels in the leg are invisible.
- Skin has to move freely over the keel.
- Birds are not supposed to "hit" the drinkers.
- Good hatchery managers pull the hatch at a time appropriate for the majority of poults. It is necessary to have a poults hatch over the shortest time possible.

Navels

- They have to be closed and dry. Open navels favour the entry of bacteria.
- Abdomen of the poult is not supposed to be mushy when picked up. This indicates a navel infection.

Brooding systems : Poults may be started successfully either on the floor or in batteries.

Facility and equipment recommended for brooding turkeys

Item	Age of Poult	
	0-4 weeks brooding	**4-8 weeks brooding**
Space	0.5-0.6 square feet per poult	1-1-¼ square feet per poult
Brooders	1 per 100 poults	(Space heaters or brooders, as needed)
Waterers	2 per 100 poults	-
Jars	1 inch per poult	1 inch per poult
Feeders *		
Trough	3 inches per poult	3 inches per poult
Round	-	3 inches per poult

* Recommendations based on linear inches of feeding space. Trough feeders provide feeding space on both sides, so a feeder of 3 feet long provides 6 feet of feeding space. Measure the outer circumference of round feeder pans to determine available space.

Floor Brooding

Preparing for Poults

Thoroughly clean, disinfect the brooder house and equipment one week before the poults arrive. Clean out old litter and accumulated manure and remove dust from sidewalls and ceilings. The entire interior should also be thoroughly washed down. Pressurized washers are especially useful for cleaning walls, ceilings and hard-to-reach areas. Water under high pressure can also be used.

Follow the cleanout with a good disinfectant spray. Disinfectants do not penetrate accumulated dirt or manure, so they are not substitute for a thorough cleaning. Rinse the house again if recommended on the disinfectant label and allow the house to dry completely. Airing the house for several days also helps to eliminate moisture in the house.

Put down 2 inches of litter, have all equipment in place and make sure it is operating properly 2 or 3 days before the poults arrive. Early preparation allows time to make necessary repairs and adjustments. Operate brooders at the proper temperature at least 24 hours before poults are delivered, to warm house and so that the thermostats can be adjusted. Feed and water have to be available, so that the poults start eating and drinking immediately after arriving.

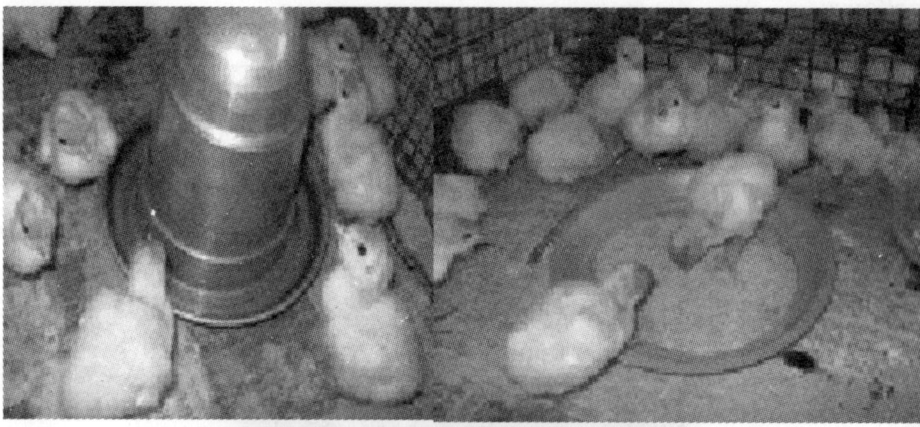

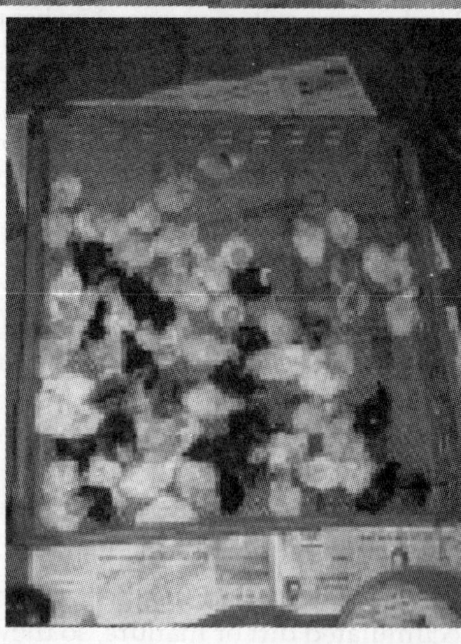

Place poults under the brooders as quietly as possible. Do not make sudden loud noises that might cause them to crowd. Check the poults quietly and frequently, especially just before and after dark.

Litter Material

Litter material has to be clean, dry, absorbent and dust-free. Paddy husk, ground nut hulls and other commercial litters can be used, depending on cost and availability. Any organic litter will support mould growth if it gets more moisture content.

Do not use excessively fine litter materials that poults are likely to consume. Litter consumption may increase mortality due to crop impaction. Litter can be covered with rough paper for the first few days to keep the poults from eating litter. Litter is not to be covered with smooth-surfaced materials since these cause serious leg problems. The paper has to be removed when the poults are 14 days old.

Remove any wet or caked litter and add new litter to maintain a depth of 5 cms. Stirring litter helps to maintain its quality as poults get older.

Brooders

Inexperienced turkey growers need not brood more than 75 to100 poults under each hover although some experienced growers may brood more. Allow at least 12 square inches of floor space per poult under hover which confine heat. Radiant brooders have smaller hovers but extend the heat area outward. Follow the manufacturer's recommendations on density for poults.

Popular brooding systems are heated by electricity or gas. Choose a system which relies on the least-costly fuel available. There is more risk of fire with open flame brooders and they are to be kept in good operating conditions.

Experienced turkey growers can select the optimum brooding temperatures by observing poults. Poults huddle together under the hover when temperature is too low and will move out against the brooder guard ring when temperature is too warm. Poults that consistently stay on one side of the brooding area are trying to escape a drafty area. Comfortable poults will spread uniformly under and around the edge of the brooder. Poults are the most accurate "thermometer", but rearers need some experience to interpret the reaction of poults.

Place a thermometer at the edge of the hover, about 7.5 cms above the litter. Brooding temperature has to be 95^0 F for the first week and lowered by 5^0 F each following week down to 75^0 F.

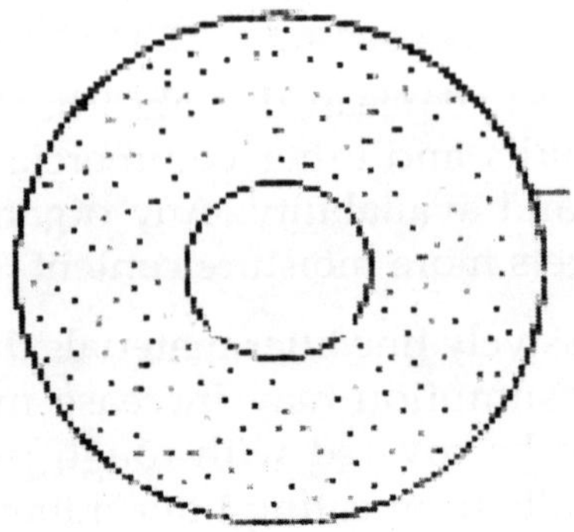

Optimum brooding temperature

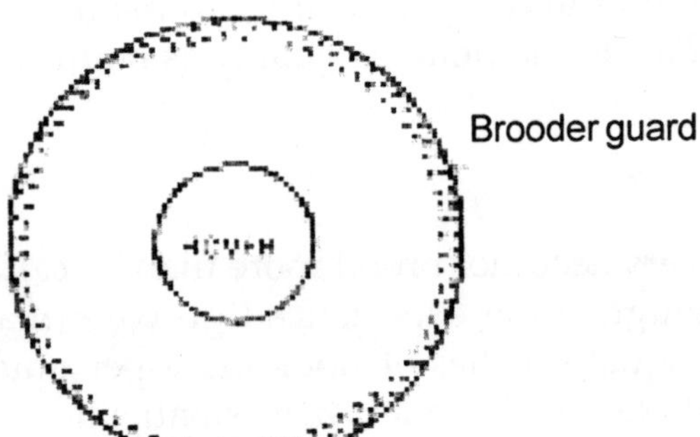

High brooding temperature

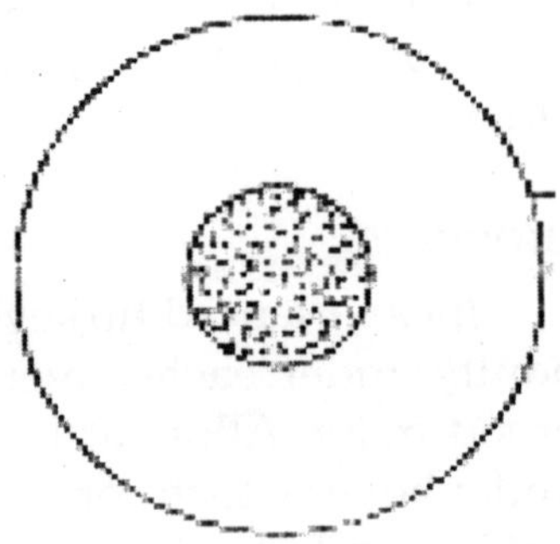

Low brooding temperature

Brooder Guards

Brooder guards are barrier placed 3 to 5 feet from the edge of the brooder to confine poults near the heat source. Guards can either be removed after a week or enlarged and retained for a second week.

Brooder guards have to be 30-45 cm high. An open mesh material (mesh as large as three-fourths of an inch) light weight hardware cloth or chicken wire can be used during warm weather. Solid materials such as metal sheets, corrugated paper, tarred paper or plywood have to be used during cold weather. The solid wall protects poults from drafts and helps retain heat near the hover area. Support the brooder guards as needed to keep them in place.

Equipments

The figure illustrates a typical initial arrangement of brooding equipment. Place feeders around the hover in a pattern resembling spokes of a wheel so feeders do not hinder movement of poults to or from the heat source. Small trays of feeder and some feeders has to be very close to the edge of the hover or extend slightly under the hover to help poults find feed. Fill water fountains and place them along the edge of the hover.

Use contrast colour tray feeders for 3-4 days, or until the poults are eating well. The trays can then be gradually removed and the feed troughs and waterers can be gradually moved away from edge of the hover. Keep the feeder troughs two third full for the first 4 days. The level of feed in troughs can then be reduced to not more than two third full to control feed wastage. After the first week, raise feeders at weekly intervals so the lip of the feeder is the same height as the poult's back. Be sure that all equipment, feed and management changes are made gradually. Proper attention is given to prevent poults from crowding or piling on top of each other in the corners of the floor pens.

Battery Brooders

Battery brooders are commonly used when smaller groups of poults are started at frequent intervals. Some growers feel the added expense of battery brooding is justified because poults get off to a good start. Poults in battery brooders can be watched closely during these critical early days of brooding. The close confinement and smaller numbers of poults per group reduce crowding problems and may help poults find feed and water earlier.

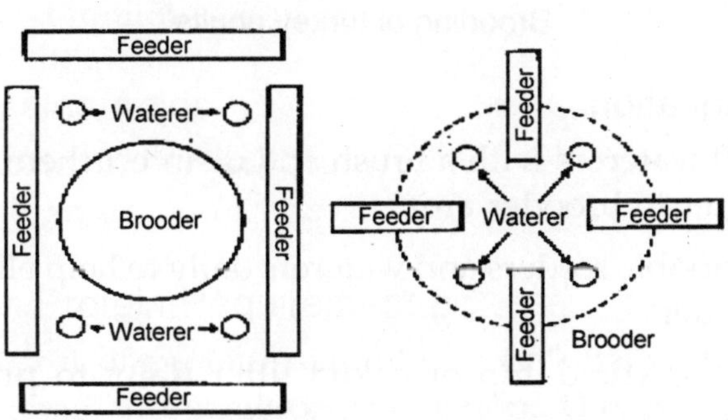

Improper arrangement of brooder Proper arrangement of brooder

Construct the battery room to provide adequate ventilation so that the room temperature can be maintained at about 70^0 F. Temperature in the warmer part of the battery has to be maintained according to the same schedule as for floor brooding. Provide 18-24 square inches of battery floor area per poult, depending on how long they stay in the battery brooder.

If the wire floor has mesh of one-half inch or larger, cover it with a coarse cloth or crinkled paper for the first few days to prevent leg injuries. Hocks frequently become caught in one-half inch wide floors. Battery brooders are heated electrically. High mortality can result from piling, especially as darkness approaches.

Light

Recommended lighting standards have generally called for relatively bright lights (10-15 foot candles) around the clock for the first 2 weeks. Thereafter, a 16-hour day is to be provided and light intensity need to be gradually reduced to 1 foot candle.

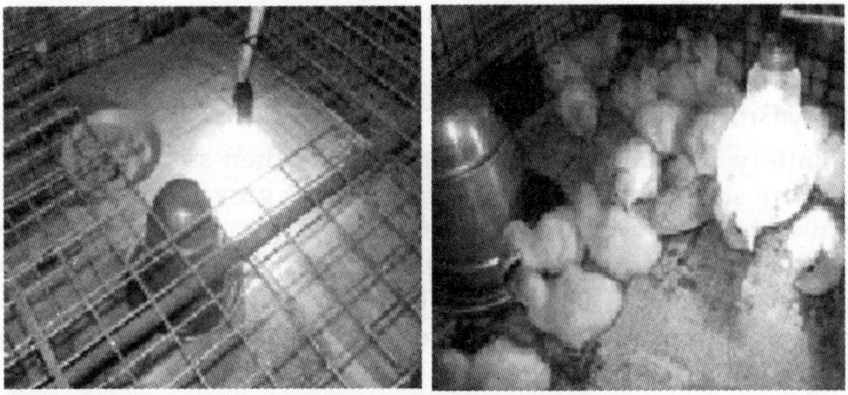

Brooding of turkey poults

Brooding Sanitation

- Clean all waterers with a brush and disinfect them daily. Do not spill water in brooder area.
- Move portable feeders and waterers daily to help eliminate damp or wet litter.
- Remove or stir damp or caked litter daily to prevent mould buildup.
- Maintain proper ventilation.
- Remove and record dead birds on each trip to the house.
- Use foot bath for disinfecting shoes and boots of caretaker at entrance of brooder house.

- Servicemen have to use disinfecting pan or keep rubber boots just inside brooder house.
- Do not allow visitors in brooder house.
- Keep all animals, rats, dogs, birds, etc. out of brooder house.

Methods to Control Mortality due to Starve out condition

Young turkey poults are not capable of taking feed properly. Therefore, in poults, starve out deaths are more common. In order to avoid this, feed can be kept in coloured plastic plates. One or two trainer chicks (chicken) can be allowed along with the turkey poults, so that the poults start taking the feed along with the chicks. Colored marbles or pebbles are placed in feeders and waterers to attract poults towards them. Since turkeys are fond of greens, some chopped green leaves can also be added to the feed to improve the feed intake. The brooder diet has to contain amino acids like lysine and methionine in required quantity. To prevent the occurrence of paralysis in turkeys, calcium and phosphorus have to be added in the diet during the first eight weeks of age.

Cannibalism

Cannibalism is one of the important vices seen in turkeys. This habit causes injury to the feathers, toes and vent.

Reasons

- Less floor space.
- Increased brooding temperature
- High energy diet
- Deficiency of salt in diet

Preventive Measures

- Proper managemental practices.
- Diet should contain adequate nutrients.

Debeaking

Debeaking controls feather picking and cannibalism. All confined birds and most range turkeys are debeaked.Debeak poults at 6-10 days of age. Commercial electrical debeakers use a red-hot iron bar to cut and cauterize the beak. Ranged turkeys can be debeaked later if picking or serious fighting occurs. Make sure feeders have at least one-half to three-fourths of feed for debeaked turkeys.

Desnooding

Desnooding removes the snood, a fleshy appendage located just behind the top of the base of the upper beak. Removing snoods of male poults reduces fighting, prevents head injuries and prevent or reduce the incidence of erysipelas. Male poults are usually desnooded at the hatchery on request of the grower.

Toe Clipping

Removal of the toenails of turkeys is usually done at the hatchery, but toes of turkeys as old as 5 weeks can be clipped when turkeys are debeaked. Toe clipping can improve the grade of processed turkeys. Turkeys in large groups, especially when excited, often step on flock mates and cause scratches or skin tears on the backs and sides. Increasing flock sizes and densities aggravate the problem, especially when turkeys are reared in confinement.

The most popular form of toe clipping involves cutting the inside and middle (front) toe on each foot. Although toes can be cut with surgical scissors or a nail clipper, a modified hot-blade debeaker cauterize the cut and reduce bleeding. Make cuts just inside of the outer toe pad to remove the root of the nail and prevent regrowth.

General Management Tips

Practice Good Husbandry

The turkey poult, like the young of any species, requires attention. Close observation of poult movement and sound reveal much about poult comfort and health. Most poult mortality can be traced to inattention, poor sanitation, infrequent visits to the brooder house, faulty equipment, inadequate ventilation, or poor husbandry.

Poults that become sick or crippled during the brooding period seldom recover fully. Injured poults have trouble in competing for feed, water and hover space. They cannot escape from being walked on or picked by other poults. Injured or sick poults usually die or develop poorly and have lower feed efficiency. Sick and crippled poults have to be destroyed since they will provide rearers with little, return.

Provide market turkeys with a complete ration, formulated to meet their nutritional needs. Provide a constant supply of fresh, clean water. Adequate feeder and waterer space is needed. Remove wet feed promptly before moulds develop. Use chlorinated water.

Visit and see flock daily and watch for sources of potential trouble such as malfunctioning equipment and dead, sick or crippled birds. Look for changes in the activity patterns of the birds. Daily records of feed and water consumption and flock mortality can be used to help spot trouble early. Check temperature regularly and adjust equipment when necessary. Clean the fans and light bulbs regularly. Air that smells bad indicates that ventilation should be improved.

A good health program prevents diseases. Good sanitation, recommended vaccination and proper use of medications are important factors in sound health programs. Accurate and early diagnosis of sick birds is a key step in controlling the spread of diseases. Commercial producers usually start several flocks each year. When turkeys are about 8 weeks old, they are moved from the brooder house to grower houses.

□□□

Chapter 5

Grower Management

Good grower management of turkeys require appropriate growth and good flock uniformity. Poor flock uniformity lead to a variable onset of egg production.

Management requirements : Floor space requirement of grower turkey

Age in weeks	Floor space (sq. feet)
9 to 12	2 - 2.5
13 to 20	3 - 3.5
21 to 24	4 - 4.5

Feeder and waterer space requirement of grower turkey

Feeding space	Watering space
5 - 7.5 cm	2.5 cm

Number of feeders and waterers required for 100 grower turkey

Age in weeks	Length of linear feeders	Number of feeders	Area of circular waterers	Number of waterers
9 to 24	120 cm	3	112 sq. cm	2

Feeding

After 8 weeks of age the turkeys are to be fed with grower mash. Feed properly balanced ration, so that they are capable of laying good number of eggs later (See chapter 7).

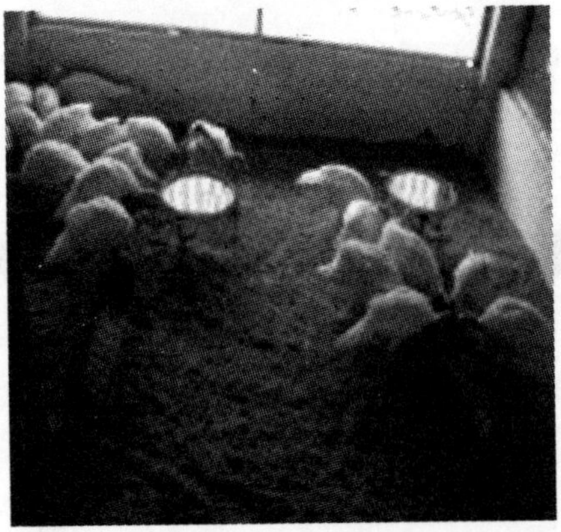

Deep litter system of rearing turkey growers

Lighting Programme

Turkeys start their reproductive cycle in response to light stimuli. For good egg production it is essential that turkey females are brought from a long day length to a short one and back again to a long day length to trigger their reproductive cycle, i.e. to mimic the natural change in day length from winter to spring.

Step Down Programme for Females During Growing

From brooding until the end of week 11 the light intensity has to be kept constant at around 30 lux, with a day length of 14 hours. It is important to check this periodically with a light meter and to clean light bulbs or tubes regularly to remove the dust that accumulates on them reducing their effectiveness. Replace always burnt out or damaged bulbs/tubes immediately. From 18 weeks of age breeder females must be reared under a short day length to ensure that they can be stimulated into egg production by an increase in day length when transferred to the laying houses. During the conditioning period, the day length is decreased to 6/7 hours and the light intensity increased to between 50 and 60 Lux.

Lighting programme for grower turkey

Ages	Hours	Lux level intensity
2 - 11	14 L : 10 D	30 lux
12	13 L : 11 D	Slowly increase from 30 lux
13	12 L : 12 D	to 50/60 lux over this period
14	11 L : 13 D	
15	10 L : 14 D	
16	9 L : 15 D	
17	8 L : 16 D	
18 - 28/29	6/7 L : 17/18 D	50 - 60 lux

Other Managemental Practices

- Growers that are stunted, crippled etc. have to be culled periodically.
- All vaccines are to be given in grower stage.
- To remove the ectoparasites, delicing is done before they start laying. If it is done after the start of lay, there will be a disruption of egg production.
- Delicing is done on the day of bright sunlight. Only after complete drying, the birds are allowed in the sheds. To prevent the birds from accidentally consuming the drug, neck of the bird has to be held and the remaining part to be immersed in the solution. For dipping malathion and sumithion can be used at the rate 0.2%.
- The birds which are grown in deep litter system have to be dewormed once in two months.
- The litter has to be raked regularly.

□□□

Chapter 6

Breeder Management

The`ultimate objective of breeding turkeys is the efficient production of quality meat. This has to be combined with a further objective of efficient chick production in the parent generation. This combination is a challenge for the primary breeder. The negative correlation which exists between these characteristics means that it is difficult to make genetic progress in both fields at the same time.

Management requirements

	Requirements
Floor space	5 sq. ft.
Feeding space	7.5 cm
Watering space	3.5 cm
Nest space / 5 hens	One nest 14 x 24 x 24 inches

Number of feeders and waterers required for 100 breeder turkeys

Age in weeks	Area of circular feeders	No. of feeders	Area of circular waterers	No. of waterers
Above 24 weeks	120 sq. cm	4	110 sq. cm	2

Sex determination

Characters	Tom	Hen
Body size	Heavy	Relatively small
Snood or dew bill	Pink/red fleshy protuberances on the head	Absent
Caruncles	Fleshy protuberance near the base of the neck; relatively large, plumb and elastic	Relatively small, thin and non-elastic
Beard	Blackish and seen in the breast region	Absent
Strut (sound produced by turkey	Sturt - day - old through to adult	Absent

Selection of Breeder Flock

The external appearance forms the basis for the selection of breeding stock. The selected birds are to be of good health and vigour. They are to be free from all diseases and disabilities. They are also to be free of defects such as crooked chest, back or legs and split wings. These defects may be transmitted to the next generation. Since the turkey is prized for its meat quality, emphasis should be placed on its dressed out appearance. Birds which have a broad breast are more preferred and such types of turkeys are mostly reared. Such broad breasted birds are called 'beef type' turkeys. Such turkeys have short neck and legs. To increase the body weight of the turkey flock; birds are to be selected at a particular age and body weight.

Nature Mating

The mating behavior of tom is known as "Strut", wherein it spreads the wings and makes a peculiar sound frequently. In natural mating the male: female ratio is 1:5 for medium type turkeys and 1:3 for large types. Toms are rarely used for mating after first year due to reduced fertility. There is a tendency in toms to develop affinity towards a particular female, so the toms have to be changed every 15 days.

The hens start laying eggs by about 24 to 28 weeks of age. The production is economical till 52 weeks of age. A hen produces 80 to 100 eggs a year. About 50 to 60 turkey poults are obtained from a hen in a year. Nearly 70 percent of the eggs are laid in the afternoon. Eggs are collected frequently to increase hatchability and eliminate the chance of floor eggs and eggs being broken in the nests.

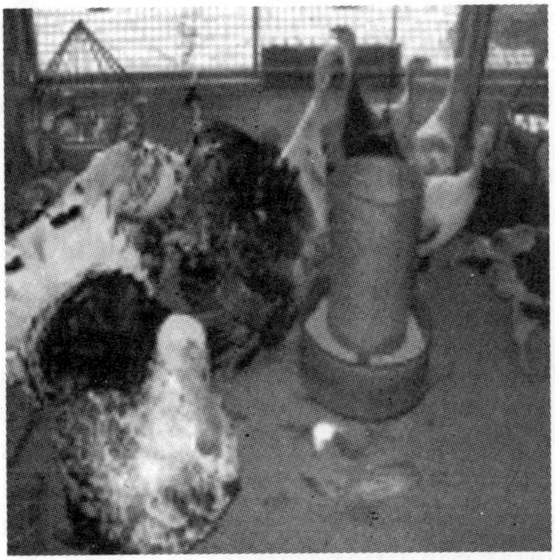

Mating

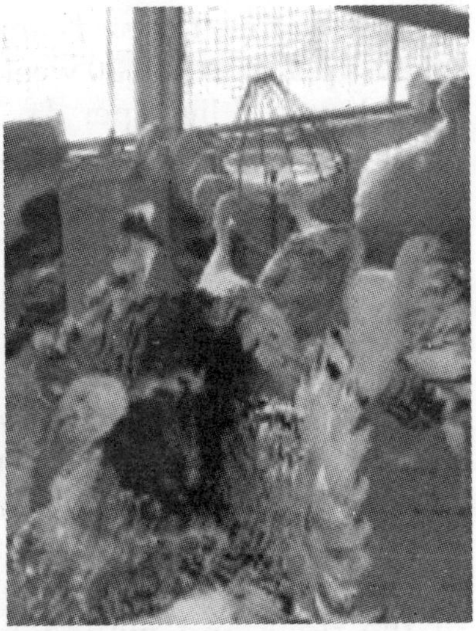

Strut

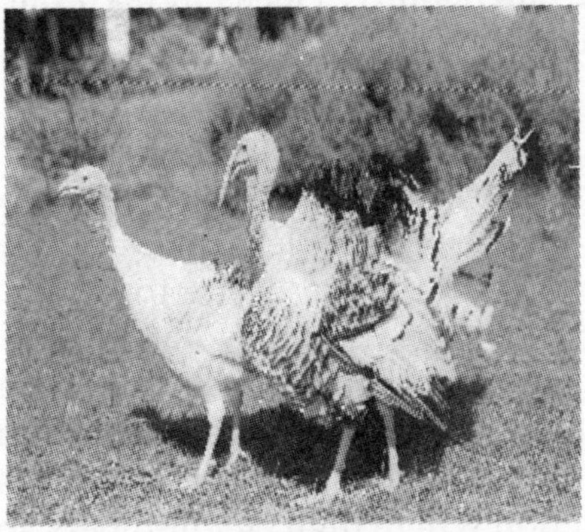

Tom and Hen Turkey

Feeding

Breeder rations have to be fortified with minerals and vitamins for obtaining better fertility and hatchability. (See chapter- 7)

Lighting

Breeder turkeys are raised under specific lighting programs. Toms are raised with 12 hours of daylight per day to ensure good semen production at the right age. Hens are raised on a normal commercial lighting program (14 hours of light per day) until 16 weeks of age. Then the lighting is reduced on a gradual basis down to 6 hours per day by the time the birds are 20 weeks of age. They are maintained at 6 hours per day until 30 week of age when they are taken up overnight to 14 hours of light per day. This is called photo stimulation, which stimulates egg production. When hens are brought into production in naturally ventilated (open or curtain sided) housing during periods of long natural day length, then this day length has to be maintained throughout the laying period.

Fertility and Hatchability

Fertility and hatchability for a flock are expressed as percentages in relation to total eggs set. Hatchability is also be expressed in percentage in relation to fertile eggs set. Varieties, strains, family as well as individuals within a family differ with respect to fertility and hatchability. Age of birds, season, light, nutritional and health status of the flock and managemental conditions affect fertility and hatchability.Very high or low temperature in the breeding house affect fertility and hence hatchability. Flocks in high rate of lay have better fertility and hatchability than poorly producing flocks.

Broody Control

In the wild, the turkey female begins to lay eggs in the spring stimulated by the increasing day length. Once hen turkey has laid a clutch of eggs (10 to 15) a natural desire to incubate them takes over and hen will sits on the eggs until they hatch some 28 days later. This is known as broody behaviour, caused by a build up of natural secretions of the hormone prolactin in the bloodstream. Once a female becomes broody it ceases to lay eggs, which is not desirable in commercial production where high egg numbers are required. Broody control describes the husbandry techniques used to prevent turkey females from becoming broody. Females should be encouraged to lay their eggs in the nest boxes, as those which lay their eggs on the floor can be more difficult to treat. Pens have to be evenly lit and designed with as few corners as possible to discourage floor layers.

Artificial Insemination in Turkeys

Artificial insemination helps in increasing fertility of the turkeys during the breeding period.

Collection of Semen from Tom

- The age of tom has to be 32-36 weeks for semen collection.

- The tom has to be kept in isolation at least 15 days before semen collection.
- The tom has to be handled regularly and the time required to collect the semen is 2 minutes.
- As the toms are sensitive to handling, the same operator has to be used to get maximum volume of semen.
- Average semen volume is 0.15 to 0.30 ml.
- Use the semen within one hour of collection.
- Collect semen thrice a week or on alternative days.

Culling of Unproductive turkeys : Characteristics for distinguishing a layer from a non layer.

External characteristics	Laying hen	Non-laying hen
Comb and wattles	Full, red, waxy, warm and velvet like	Dry, hard, cold, coarse and shrunken with white scabs.
Caruncles	The carungles are shiny and soft	The caruncles are dry
Beak	Stocky, well curved, worn out and less yellow	Very long, thin and sharp pointed, yellow
Eyes	Bright and alert	Dull and sleepy
Ear-lobes	Full, waxy and velvet like	Shrunken, wrinkled and coarse
Pelvic bones	Wide apart, usually spread more than 2 fingers, thin and pliable	Practically close together, thick and stiff
Abdomen	Large, spread 3 to 5 fingers soft and less of fat	Small, usually less than 2 fingers, hard and more of fat
Crop	Nearly always full	May or may not be full
Vent	Full, large and moist	Small, dry and puckered

Insemination in Hens

- Artificial insemination is done when the flock attains 8-10% egg production.

Diagram of a Tom and Hen Turkey

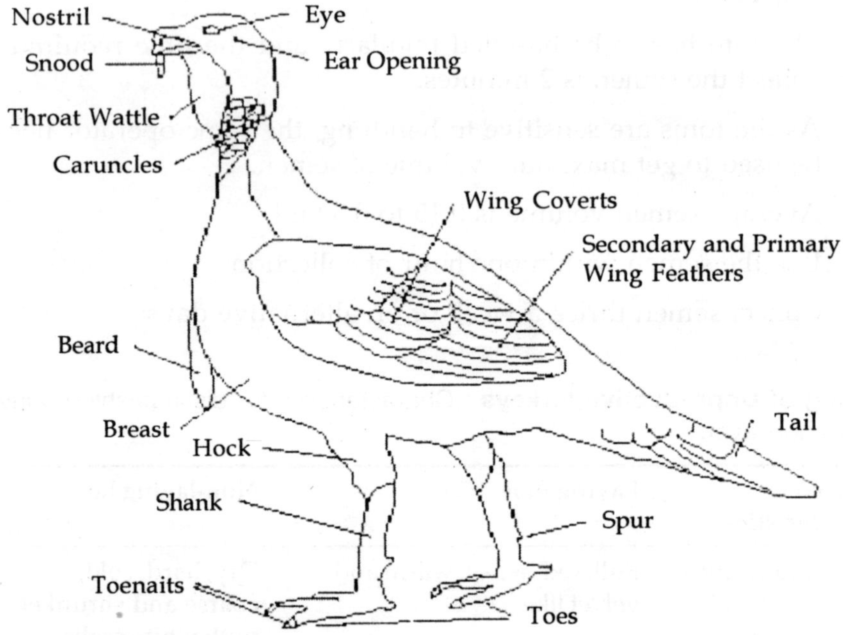

Male Turkey (Tom)

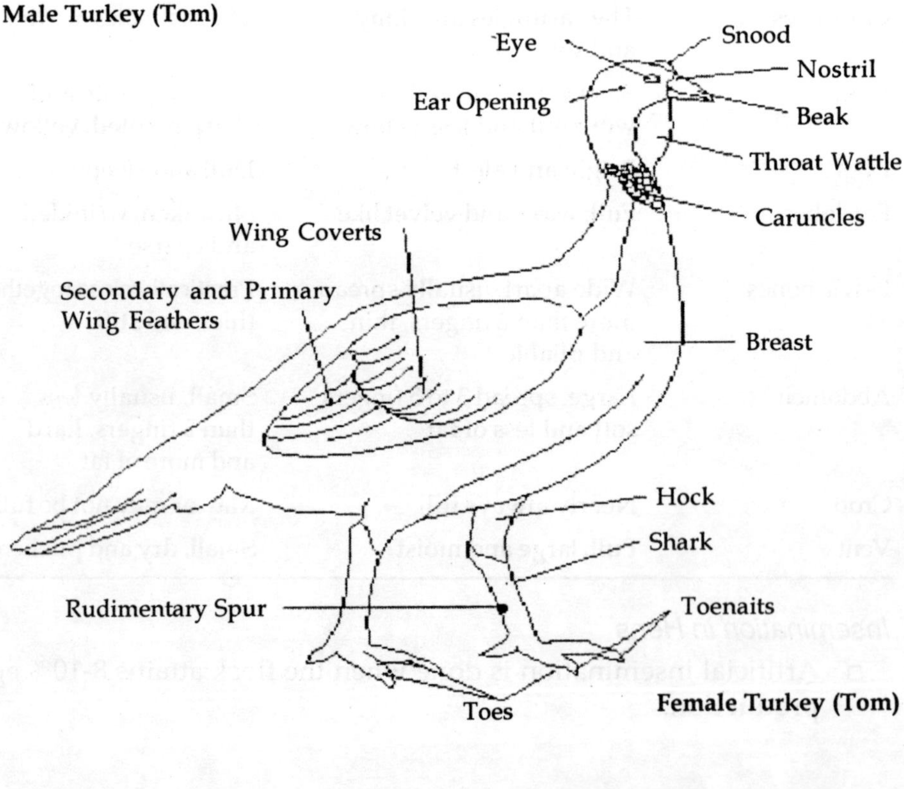

Female Turkey (Tom)

- Inseminate the hens every three weeks with 0.025-0.030 ml of undiluted semen.
- After 12 weeks of laying it is better to inseminate every fortnight.
- Inseminate the hen in the evening.
- The average fertility should be 80-85% over a 16 week breeding season.

□□□

Chapter 7

Feeding Management

The quality of turkey poults, management and disease resistance of the turkeys together determine the productivity of the turkeys. Even though the managemental practices are good, if optimal nutrients are not provided, the expected growth and productivity do not occur. For better growth of turkey poults, higher level of crude protein, minerals and vitamins are required than broilers. Turkeys require more of vitamin A, D, niacin and choline than broilers.

Feeding and Disease Resistance

Disease resistance is an important part in turkey rearing. The disease resistance in birds also varies according to the nutrient content in feed. Protein should be present in required quantity. Vitamin A and E should also be present in sufficient quantities, especially; when some fungal toxins are present in the feed; as these toxins reduce the disease resistance of the birds and make them more susceptible to diseases.

Feeding and Hatchability

In hatcheries, the quality of the turkey poults produced depends upon the nutrient content of the feed of the breeders. For quality chicks to be produced, the breeders are to be fed with sufficient crude protein, vitamins and minerals.

Feeding Turkey Poults (0 to 8 weeks)

The nutrient requirement of male and female turkey poults vary and hence it is advisable to separate male and females immediately after hatching.

Immediately after hatching, the poults are to be provided with feed. Feed is to be provided at least four times a day. The feed for turkey poults are to be kept in a place with good lighting facility. For first day, feed can be spread over the newspaper. Thereafter feed should be kept in plastic plates. For first four weeks, the feed provided has to contain 28% crude protein and 2800 k cal of energy. From 4 to 8 weeks of age, the feed has to contain 26% crude protein and 2800 k cal energy.

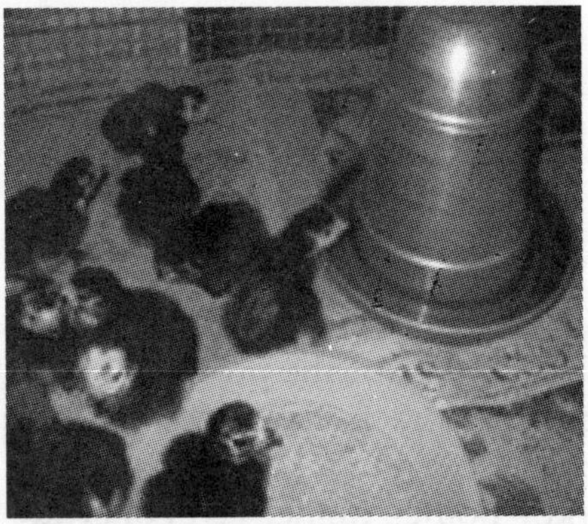

Feeding turkey poults

Feeding Turkey Growers (9 to 24 weeks)

Turkey grower feed has to contain a crude protein content of 21% crude protein, and 2700 k cal of energy.

Feeding Turkey Breeders (after 24 weeks)

Breeder turkeys have to be provided with 14% crude protein and 2600 k cal energy. The feed given to turkey males has to contain only 12-13% crude protein.

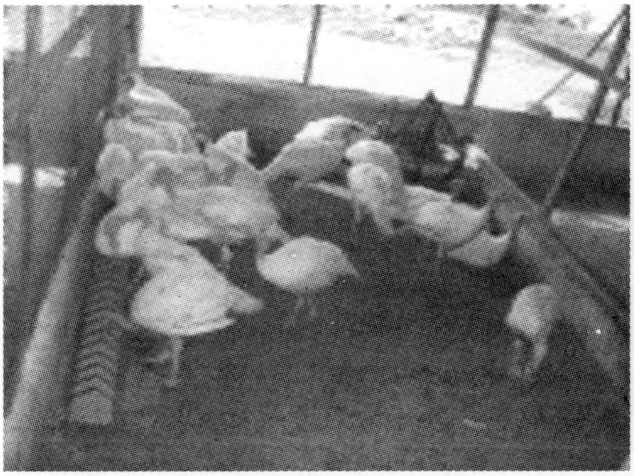

Feeding turkey growers

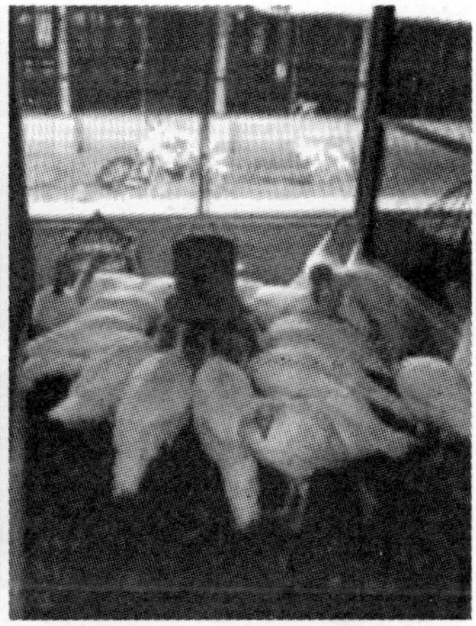

Feeding turkey breeders

Methods to Reduce Cost of Rearing in Turkeys

Green Leaves Feeding

In intensive system, green leaves can be fed upto 50% of the total diet on dry mash basis. Fresh Lucerne is first class green feed for turkeys of all ages. Apart from this Desmanthus and Stylo can be chopped and given to turkeys to reduce the feed cost.

Nutrient requirements of turkey

Nutrients	**Turkey prebrooder mash (0 to 4 weeks)**	**Turkey brooder mash (5 to 8 weeks)**	**Turkey grower mash (9 to 24 weeks)**	**Turkey breeder mash (above 24 weeks)**
Metabolizable energy (Kcal/kg)	2800	2800	2700	2600
Crude protein (%)	28.00	26.00	21.00	14.00
Calcium (%)	1.30	1.10	1.00	2.30
Phosphorus (%)	1.00	0.50	0.45	0.40
Lysine (%)	1.70	1.60	1.20	1.00
Methionine (%)	0.50	0.50	0.40	0.40

Chapter 8

Summer and Winter Management

Turkeys are susceptible to high temperature and cold. During the months of April, May and June the environmental temperature remains high; as a result, the temperature with in the house increases, which in turn cause stress to the birds. The optimum temperature and relative humidity inside the house has to be 75°F and 60-70%; respectively. Although most places are affected by a rise in temperature, the costal areas where both the temperature and relative humidity high are the most affected.

Effects of High Temperature

When the birds are 'heat stressed' they have difficulty in achieving a balance between body heat production and body heat loss. As the temperatures increases, the rate of panting increases (method of heat loss). If heat production becomes greater than 'maximum heat loss' either in intensity (acute heat stress) or over long periods (chronic heat stress), birds die (Heat stroke). The body temperature of the birds must remain very close to 41°C (106°F). If body temperature rises more than 2-4°C above this, the birds die.

When the environmental temperature increases, feed intake decreases and water intake increases. There is a decrease in egg production because of lower feed intake. In addition, the thickness of the egg shell also decreases resulting in the formation of leathery eggs. The quality of the egg albumin and yolk decreases, therefore the chances of spoilage of stored egg increases. During peak summer the infestations caused by lice, ticks and other ectoparasites are also high. When humidity and temperature are high, the occurrence of coccidiosis is also be more.

Measures to Prevent Heat Stress

- Clean, sanitized drinking water has to be made available to the birds continuously.
- Provide feed during the cooler parts of the day.
- Optimal floor space has to be provided.
- The roof can be painted with white paint so that a reduction in temperature can be achieved in the shed.
- Paddy straw, dried Palmyra or Coconut leaves can be spread over the roof which helps to reduce the temperature.
- Sprinklers can be used to sprinkle water over the roof which helps in reducing the temperature.
- Foggers can also be used in cage houses.
- The mesh has to be cleaned regularly so that there is no hindrance in ventilation and air flow which further helps in the reduction of the temperature.
- During summer, the feed intake decreases and the energy requirement of the birds also decreases. So the amount of nutrient intake has to be adjusted by increasing the nutrient density of the feed.
- Trees can be planted in and around the shed, so that it provides shade to the birds.

Winter Management

The winter season is from October to February in India. Turkey poults of 1 to 5 weeks old are the ones which are most vulnerable.

Management During Winter Season

- Artificial heat can be provided.
- Care should be taken to avoid huddling. This causes stampede of poults resulting in mortality.
- The sides of the shed can be closed using curtains or gunny bags as this minimizes the loss of heat from the house and prevent seepage of rain water inside the sheds.
- During winter, in order to maintain constant body temperature the feed intake of the birds increases. The feed provided during this season has to contain more energy.

□□□

Chapter 9

Flock Health and Biosecurity

When there is low threshold level of management of turkeys or when the disease resistance is low, there are chances of the birds to be infected. But, for certain diseases, turkeys are more resistant than chicken. The mortality suffered by most turkey flock is high in the first two weeks of age. Reasons for mortality is significantly due to "starve-outs" and yolk sac infections. Some of the other causes of mortality apart from diseases are cold shock, drug toxicity and poor ventilation.

Etiology

- Pathogenic microorganisms (viruses, bacterial and fungi) and parasites
- Nutritional deficiencies
- Metabolic disorders
- Environment

Transmission of Infectious Diseases

- Contagious from diseased or carrier birds
- Contagious from insects, rodents, and free-flying birds
- Airborne
- Contact with contaminated materials (e.g. litter, feed)
- Egg transmission
- Carcasses of dead birds that have not been disposed of properly
- Contaminated water source

Signs of Disease

- Reduced intake of feed and water
- Low rate of growth/egg production
- Abnormal droppings
- Abnormal physiological indicators: temperature >107° F, pulse rate of >400 per minute and rate of breathing of >36 per minute
- General droopiness and ruffled feathers

Measures to Prevent Disease Outbreak

- Application of a stringent quarantine program
- The control of vehicles and visitors to the farm
- Good quality poults should be procured from hatchery
- Poults are not be bought from a breeder farm which is affected by diseases
- Feed and water supplied to the birds should be hygienic
- There has to be no water logging in sheds during rainy season
- Vaccinations are to be done for the diseases which are prevalent in the region
- Deworming to be done once in two months to remove the endo parasites
- Dipping to be done to remove the ecto parasites
- The use of a preventive medication program
- The birds which show the symptoms of disease are to be isolated and treatment has to be started immediately

- Post mortem has to be performed to identify the exact cause and necessary steps should be taken to avoid the spread of the disease
- Dead birds and unhatched eggs are to be removed immediately and buried or burned
- The sheds are to be rodent proof
- After the sale of each batch of turkeys, the litter and other wastes have to be removed and the shed is to be disinfected properly
- The use of monitoring procedures to keep a check on the disease organism status of the farm, to check on the effectiveness of cleaning and sanitation procedures and to test the immunity levels to certain diseases in the stock to check the effectiveness of the vaccination program

Measures to be Taken During Outbreak

- Quick disposal of dead birds.
- All sanitation measures of drinking water to be adopted.
- Spraying of disinfectant in the shed.
- Separation of working personnel of infected pen from healthy pens.
- Personnel hygiene before and after entering in the infected pens.
- Use Vitamin E and C to overcome stress.
- Frequent change of infected litter.
- Quick separation and disposal of sick and ailing birds.

Measures to be Taken After Breakout

- Infected flock after recovery to be disposed off quickly.
- Emptied sheds and infected equipment are to be thoroughly cleaned and disinfected before reusing the same.
- Disinfected sheds can be kept empty for 2-3 weeks before housing the birds.
- Infected litter has to be burned or buried properly.

Vaccination Schedule

Day Old	ND-B1 Strain
4-5 Week	Fowl Pox
6th Week	ND - (R2B)
8-10 Week	Cholera Vaccine

Common Diseases of Turkey

	Cause	Symptoms	Prevention
Arizonosis	*Salmonella arizona*	Poults unthirfty and may develop eye opacity and blindness. Susceptible age 3 - 4 weeks	Elimination of infected brrder flock and hatchery fumigation and sanitation.
Blue comb disease	*Corona virus*	Depression, loss of weight, frothy or watery droppings, darkening of head and skin.	Depopulation and decontamination of farm. Give rest period.
Chronic respiratory disease	*Mycoplasma gallisepticum*	Coughing, gurgling, sneezing, nasal exudates	Secure *Mycoplasma* free stock
Erysipelas	*Erysipelothrix rhusiopathidae*	Sudden losses, swollen snood, discoloration of parts of face, droppy	Vaccination
Fowl cholera	*Pasturella multocida*	Purplish head, greenish yellow droppings, sudden death	Sanitation and disposal of dead birds.
Fowl pox	*Pox virus*	Small yellow blisters on comb and wattles and scab formation	Vaccination
Haemorrhagic enteritis	*Virus*	One or more dead birds	Vaccination
Infectious synovitis	*Mycoplasma gallisepticum*	Enlarged hocks, foot pads, lameness, breast blisters	Purchase clean stock
Infectious sinusitis	*Bacteria*	Nasal discharge, swollen sinuses and coughing	Secure poults from disease free breeders
Mycotoxicosis	*Fungal origin*	Haemorrhages, pale, fatty liver and kidneys	Avoid feed spoilage
New castle disease	*Paramyxo Virus*	Gasping, wheezing, twisting of neck, paralysis, soft shelled eggs	Vaccination
Paratyphoid	*Salmonella pullorum*	Diarrhea in pouls	Prevention and flock sanitation

Turkey coryza	*Bordetella avium*	Snicking, rales and discharge of excessive nasal mucus	Vaccination
Coccidiosis	*Coccidia spp*	Bloody diarrhea and loss of weight	Proper sanitation and management of litter
Turkey venereal disease	*Mycoplasma meleagris*	Lowered fertility and hatchability	Strict sanitation

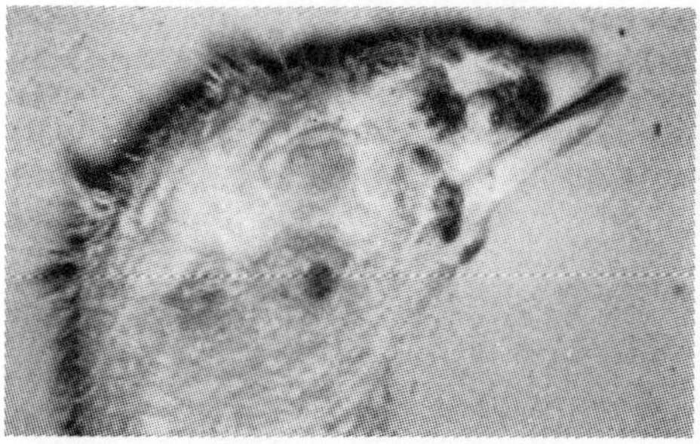

Fowl pox - Small yellow pustules on comb and wattles

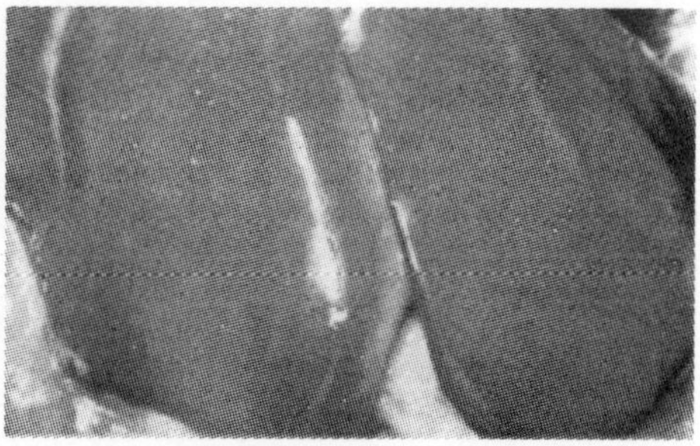

Fowl cholera - Liver

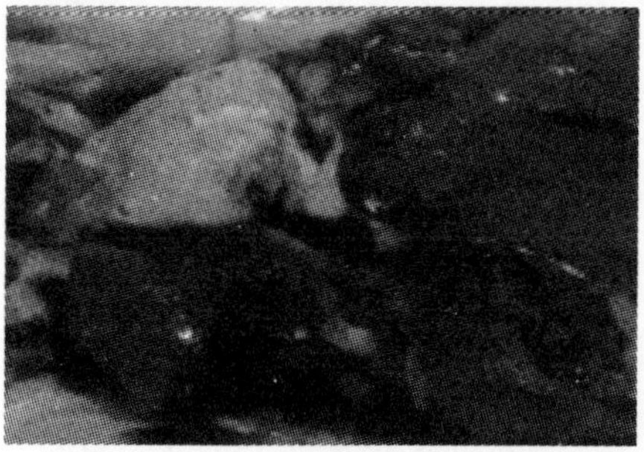

Liver

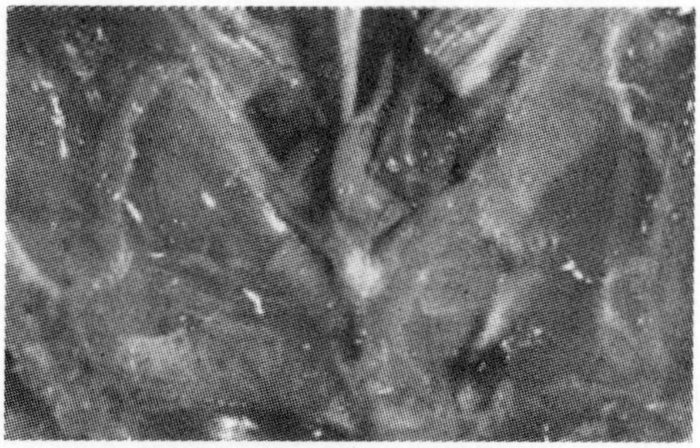

Lungs and airsac

Chronic respiratory disease

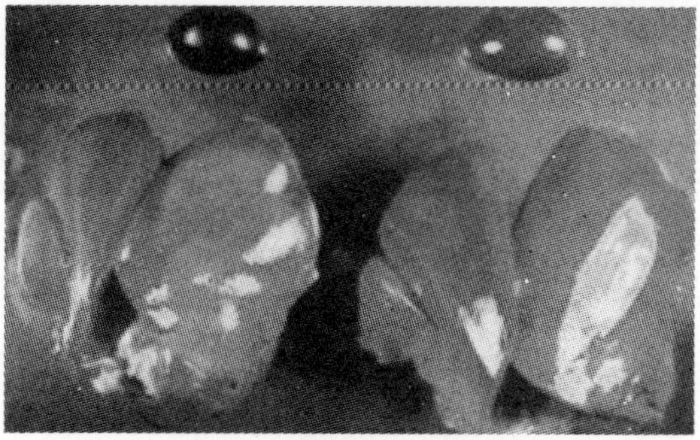

Fowl typhoid - Liver

□□□

Chapter 10

Nutritive Value of Egg and Meat and Its Processing

Turkey Egg

Turkey egg is considered to be one of the best sources of animal protein.

Turkey Meat

The turkey meat is low fat, high protein compared with red meat and is therefore a good raw material for products to be made for an increasingly sedentary and informed consumer. The protein, fat, energy value of turkey meat is 20 g, 7.77 g, 157 calories per 100 gm of meat; respectively. An average portion of turkey meat (100g) provides 20 g of protein, approximately half a woman's daily requirement and almost half a man's requirement. Mineral like potassium, calcium, magnesium, iron, selenium, zinc and sodium are present. It is also rich in essential amino acids and vitamins like niacin, vitamin B6 and B12. It is rich in unsaturated fatty acids and essential fatty acids and low in cholesterol. The dressing percentage turkey is 72% with yield of breast - 32%, thigh and legs - 32%, wings - 15% and back - 21%.

Nutritive value of turkey egg - fresh (raw)

Amount - 1 egg (79 g)

Calories : 135 Carbohydrate : 0.91 g Protein : 10.81 g Fat : 9.39 g

Vitamin A - 438IU	Calcium - 78 mg
Vitamin B1 (Thiamin) - 0.09 mg	Iron - 3.24 mg
Vitamin B2 (Riboflavin) - 0.37 mg	Magnesium - 10 mg
Vitamin B3 (Niacin) - 0.02 mg	Phosphorus - 134 mg
Vitamin B5 (Pantothenic Acid) - 1.49 mg	Potassium - 112 mg
Vitamin B6 (Pyridoxine) - 0.1 mg	Sodium - 119 mg
Vitamin B12 (Cobalamin) - 1.34 mcg	Zinc - 1.25 mg
Folate - 56 mcg	Copper - 0.05 mg
Vitamin C - 0 mg	Manganese - 0.03 mg
Vitamin D - 0 IU	Fluoride - 0 mcg
Vitamin E - 0 mg	Selenium - 27.1 mcg
Vitamin K - 0 mcg	

Composition of poultry meat

Nutrient	Turkey	Duck	Quail	Chicken
Protein (g)	20.37	11.49	19.63	18.33
Total fat 9g)	7.77	39.34	12.05	14.83
Carbohydrate (g)	0.08	0.0	1.20	0.13
Energy (Kcal)	157.0	404.0	192.0	213.0

Fat and protein content in turkey meat (100 g)

Nutrient	Calories	Total fat	Protein
Breast with skin	194	8 g	29 g
Breast with out skin	161	4 g	30 g
Wing with skin	238	13 g	27 g
Leg with skin	213	11 g	28 g
Dark meat with skin	232	13 g	27 g
Dark meat with out skin	192	8 g	28 g
Skin only	482	44 g	19 g

Steps in Processing Turkeys

Processing is the changing of the natural/normal raw product into convenient ready-to work/cook products.

- Suspend by legs in a steel shackle.
- Stunning.
- Bleeding.
- Scalding.
- Feather removal (Picking).
- Evisceration.
- Chilling.
- Packaging.
- Further processing.

Further Processing

Further processing is the adding of value to the raw product either by pre-cooking, crumbing or the adding of marinates. The reasons for the development of easy to prepare or ready to eat products are the advantages for both the producer and the consumer:

Producer

- Producing high quality products
- Use lower grade raw material

Cut up parts

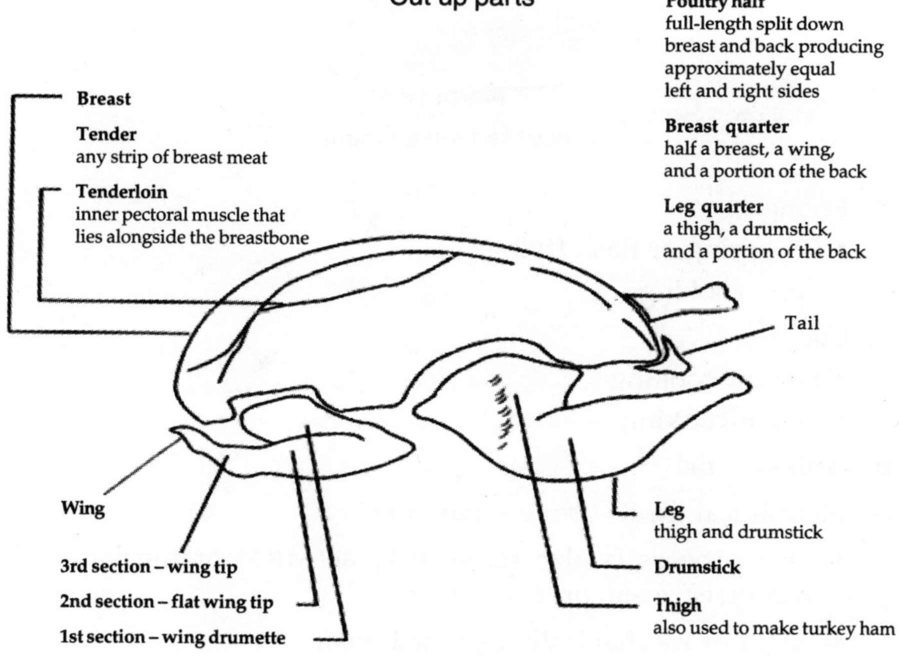

- Portion weight control
- Simple processing method
- More product variety

Consumer

- Cheaper products
- Easy to prepare
- No waste at preparation
- Short cooking time

The basic processes for adding value are:

- Forming
- Coating
  - Pre dusting
  - Battering
  - Breading or crumbing

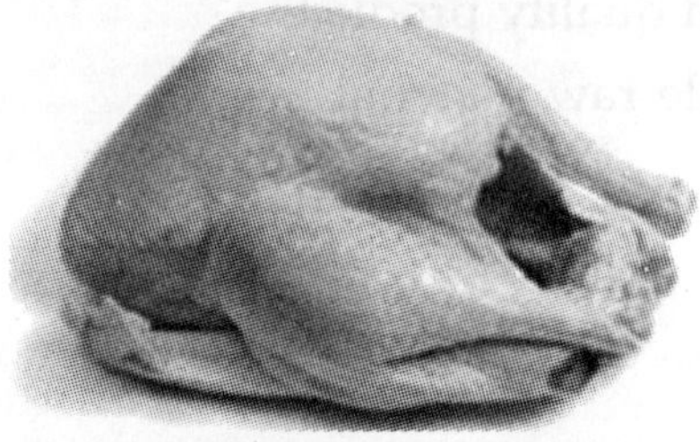

Processed turkey meat

- Frying
  - Pre-frying or flash frying
  - Fully cooking
- Cooking
  - Hot air cooking
  - Steam cooking
- Grill systems
- Mechanical meat - bone separators
  - This process is also referred to as MRM or mechanically recovered meat, or
  - MDM or mechanically deboned meat

Some of the further processed products available in North America

- Turkey ham and smoked ham,
- Deli sliced turkey, turkey ham and smoked turkey,
- Turkey bacon with alternating white and dark meats
- Mechanically de-boned turkey meat,
- Ground turkey meat products such as turkey hamburger, sausage,
- Ground turkey meat products in an emulsion e.g., frankfurters.

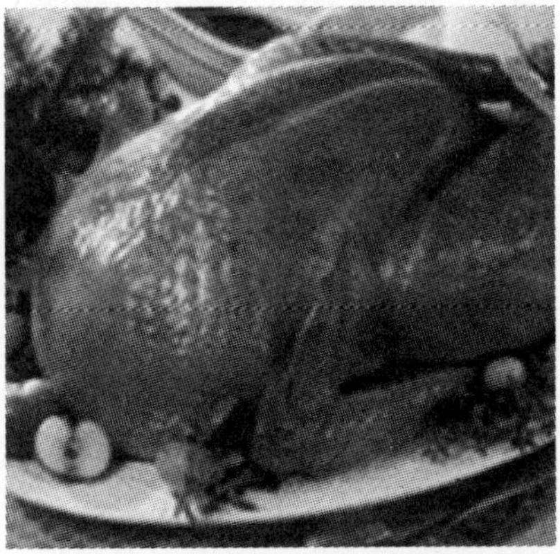

Value added turkey meat

□□□

Chapter 11

Marketing and Economics

Marketing

The marketing of turkeys has been confined largely to the festive season during the months of November, December and January. There has been a definite trend during the past few years to extend the marketing of turkeys over a longer period. Turkeys are ready for market when they are 16 to 24 weeks of age, since it is not economical to feed turkeys beyond this period. There is an increase in the quantity of feed required to produce a kilogram of turkey after about 20 weeks of age. The absolute gains in weight during the later stages of growth are large, but in terms of cost these gains are also the most expensive. The average body weight is 4-6 Kgs and the birds are generally lifted by the traders from the farm. There appears to be no retail market for the birds on day to day basis except during festive season like Christmas, Deepavali etc.

The Indian turkey market remains primarily a live bird market. Although there is a growing trend in consumption of chilled and frozen turkey products in restaurants, most consumers prefer fresh turkey meat. Birds for home consumption are typically purchased live and slaughtered in poultry retail shops. Demand for frozen turkey products will continue to remain constrained by inadequate cold chain facilities. Luxury hotels account for most of the consumption of processed turkey products such as sausages, salami, etc.

Economics of Turkey Farming (100 Turkeys)

Assumptions

Cost of day old poult	Rs. 60/-
Cost of feed/kg	Rs. 18/kg
Average feed consumption/bird (upto 24 wks)	16 kg
Space requirement per bird	4 sq. ft
Medication and vaccinations	Rs. 10/turkey
Cost of construction of shed	Rs. 75 /sq feet
Equipments	Rs. 15/turkey
Market age	24 weeks
Average market weight in kg (24 weeks)	4 kg
Mortality (24 weeks)	5%
Sale price: Live	Rs. 120/kg
Dressed	Rs. 200/kg

I. Fixed Cost

Construction of turkey shed (100 poults- 400 sq. ft.)	Rs. 30,000/-
Equipment costs (100 poults)	Rs. 1500/-
Total	**Rs. 31,500/-**

II. Recurring Cost

Cost of turkey poults	Rs. 6000/-
Feed cost (97.5 turkeys; mid point mortality)	Rs. 28,080/-
Medicine and vaccination cost	Rs. 1,000/-
Total	**Rs. 35,080/-**

III Gross Return

Sale of 95 turkeys (5% total mortality)	Rs. 45, 600/-

IV. Gross Profit

Gross Return - Recurring Cost	Rs. 10,520/-
Profit per bird sold	Rs. 105/-
Profit per kg sold	Rs. 26/-

❑❑❑

Chapter 12

Bank Loan and Insurance

In order to obtain bank loan the farm(ers) have to apply to the nearest branch of a Commercial or Cooperative or Regional Rural Banks in their area in the prescribed application forms which is available in the branches of financing banks. The technical officers attached to or the manager of the bank can give guidance to the farmers in preparing the project report to obtain bank loan.

For poultry farming projects with very large outlays, detailed reports will have to be prepared. Banks provide financial assistance for the following purposes:

- For construction of brooder/grower and layer sheds, feed store, quarters etc.
- For purchase of poultry equipment such as feeders, waterer, brooders etc.
- For creating infrastructure items for supply of electricity, feed, water etc.

- For purchase of day old chicks or ready to lay pullets.
- For meeting working capital requirement in respect of feed, medicines and veterinary aid etc. for the first 5 to 6 months (i.e. till the stage of income generation).

However, if land is purchased for establishing a poultry farm, land cost can be treated as party's margin upto a maximum of 10% of total cost of project.

Project Report Formulation for Bank Loan

A project can be prepared by the beneficiary after consulting local technical persons of State Veterinary department, Poultry Corporation or University. If possible, they can also visit the progressive turkey farms in the area and discuss the profitability of farming. A good practical training and experience on a turkey farm is highly desirable, before starting a farm. A regular and constant demand for meat and nearness of the farm to the market should be ensured.

The project should include information on land, water and electricity facility, marketing aspects, training facilities and experience of entrepreneurs and the type of assistance available from State government, Poultry Corporation, local hatcheries. It can also include data on proposed capacity of the farm, total cost of the project, margin money to be provided by the beneficiary, requirement of bank loan, estimated annual expenditure, income and profit and the period for repayment of loan and interest.

Requirements of a Good Project

After the scheme is submitted to the bank it is examined for technical feasibility and economic viability.

A. Technical Feasibility

This briefly include:

- Suitability of climate and potentiality of the area
- Availability of inputs such as chicks, feed, medicines etc.
- Technical norms
- Infrastructure available for veterinary aid, marketing, training and experience of the beneficiary.

B. Financial Viability

This briefly include

- Unit cost and loan requirement.
- Input costs for chicks, feed, veterinary aid, labour and other overheads.
- Output costs i.e. sale of eggs, culled birds, for meat, manure, empty gunny bags etc.
- Income-expenditure statement and annual gross surplus.
- Cash flow analysis.
- Repayment schedule i.e. repayment of principal loan amount and interest.

Scrutiny of Project by the Bank

After the scheme is submitted to the bank it is examined for technical feasibility and economic viability. Other documents such as loan application forms, security aspects, margin money requirement etc. are also examined. A field visit to scheme area is undertaken for conducting techno economic feasibility study for appraisal of the scheme.

Sanction of Bank Loan and its Allocation

After ensuring technical feasibility and financial viability the scheme is sanctioned by the bank. The loan is allocated in 2 or 3 stages against the creation of specific assets such as construction of sheds, purchase of equipment and machinery, recurring cost during growing period on purchase of first batch of chicks, feed, medicines and vaccines, electricity and water, labour expenses etc. Constant follows up and supervision of the scheme is done by the bank.

Lending Terms-General

Unit Cost

Each Regional Office (RO) of NABARD has constituted a State Level Unit Cost Committee under the Chairmanship of RO in charge and with the members from developmental agencies, commercial banks and cooperative banks to review the unit cost of various investments once in six months.

Margin Money

NABARD has defined farmers into three different categories and where subsidy is not available the minimum down payment as shown below is collected from the beneficiaries.

S. No.	Category of farmer	Farmer level of predevelopment return to resources	Beneficiary's contribution
a)	Small farmers	Upto Rs. 11, 000	5 %
b)	Medium farmers	Rs. 11, 001 to Rs. 19, 250	10 %
c)	Large farmers	Above Rs. 19, 251	15 %

Interest Rate

As per the RBI guidelines issued from time to time.

Interest rate

Size of credit limit	Repayable upto 3 years	Repayable in 3 years and above
Upto Rs. 50, 000/-	8.5 %	9 %
Over Rs. 50, 000/- upto Rs. 2 lacs	9.5 %	9.75 %
Over Rs. 2 lacs upto rs. 5 lacs	10.25 %	10.25 %
Over Rs. 5 lacs upto Rs. 25 lacs	11.25 %	11.75 %
Over Rs. 25 lacs based on credit risk assessment	10.75 % to 12.25 %	11.25 % to 12.75 %

Security to be furnished

Amount of loan	Security to be furnished
A. Where movable assets are not created (eg. Dugwells, development of land etc.)	
a) Upto Rs. 10, 000/-	a) Personal Guarantee
b) Above Rs. 10, 000/-	b) i. Personal Guarantee ii. Mortgage of land
B. Where movable assets are created (pump set, pipeline etc.)	
a) Upto Rs. 50, 000/-	a) Hypothecation of the asset created
b) Above Rs. 50, 000/- to Rs. 1 lac	b) i. Hypothecation of the asset created ii. Mortgage of land or thir party guarantee
c) Above Rs. 1 lac	c) i. Hypothecation of the assets created ii. Mortage of land

Security

Security will be as per NABARD/RBI guidelines issued from time to time.

Repayment of Loan

Repayment period depends upon the gross surplus in the scheme. The loan will be repaid in suitable monthly/quarterly installments usually within a period of seven to eight years with first year as grace period.

Documents to be Produced by the Applicant

- Certified copies of records in respect of lands owned/leased.
- NOC/No Due Certificate from other financial institutions wherever applicable.
- Two passport size photographs.
- Documents of title and other relevant documents, wherever landed properties are taken as security.
- Plan and estimate in respect of construction/drilling/deepening of wells, proforma invoice/quotations in case of machines, vehicle, etc.
- Valuation certificate of the land from a competent authority/ panel valuer wherever applicable.
- Other documents related to specific schemes.

Poultry Insurance Scheme

- Thre are comprehensive insurance schemes available with the General Insurance firms applicable to poultry farms consisting layer birds, broiler birds and parent stock (Hatchery) which are exotic and cross-bred.
- All birds in a farm has to be covered. After issuing policy, if additional birds are introduced in the farm, immediate notice to be given to insurer otherwise claim will be repudiated.
- The schemes are applicable to poultry farms consisting of minimum number of birds as specified.
- The schemes are available for insuring birds in the following age groups.

Broilers	:	1 day to 8 weeks
	:	1 day to 6 weeks
Layers	:	1 day to 20 weeks
	:	21 weeks to 72 weeks
	:	1 day to 72 weeks
Hatchery Birds (Parent Stock)	:	1 day to 72 weeks

- The premium rates are applicable on per cent basis which are applicable to the peak value of birds in the applicable categories.
- The sum insured is the peak value and for broilers is Rs 45 and for layers is Rs 75. There is a week wise valuation table in-built in the policy which is applied for calculating indemnity. In case of parent stock the same is negotiable.
- The policy is charactersied by excess and final indemnity is restricted to 80% (60% in case of Gumboro).

Insurance Coverage

The Policy provides indemnity against death of birds due to accident (including fire, lightning, flood, cyclone/storm/tempest/earthquake, strike, riot, act of terrorism) or diseases contracted or occurring during the period of insurance subject to the exclusions.

Major Exclusions

- Malicious/willful injury, neglect.
- Transit by any mode of transport.
- Improper management (including over crowding) i.e. when the farm is not run on scientific poultry management guidelines and standards laid down by Poultry Corporations/Animal Husbandry Department in regard to housekeeping, watering, feeding, vaccination, deworming, debeaking, lighting/heating, culling etc.
- Loss/death due to natural mortality, non-specified or unknown diseases or reasons.
- Undergrowth, cannibalism, action or predators like preying birds and carnivorous animal.
- Theft and clandestine sale of birds.

- Intentional slaughter of the birds except in cases where destruction is necessary to terminate incurable suffering on humane consideration and to protect remaining healthy flock to reduce additional losses on the basis of certificate issued by qualified Vet. Surgeon or in cases where destruction is resorted to by order of lawfully constituted authority, under intimation to Insurance Company.
- Consequential loss however caused.
- Permanent and partial disablement of any nature.
- Loss of production i.e. the failure due to any reasons whatsoever to lay required number of eggs or small sized eggs in layers or to attain proper weight at a particular age in Broilers.
- Marek's disease, Ranikhet disease, Fowl Pox and Infectious Bronchitis. These diseases are covered by the policy if the birds are successfully inoculated against these diseases and the necessary veterinary certificate to that effect is supplied to the company. Coccidiosis and other diseases are covered only if preventive and curative measures are taken from time to time.
- Malnutrition/shortage of water, death due to starvation because of non supply of feed to birds or similar reasons of whatsoever nature.
- Undergrowth.
- Cannibalism.
- Loss due to huddling and/or piling of birds.
- Avian leucosis Complex (A.L.C.)
- War, invasion, act of foreign enemy, hostilities (whether war be declared or not), civil war, rebellion, revolution, insurrection, mutiny, tumult, military or usurped power or any consequences thereof or attempt threat.
- Any accident, loss, destruction, damage or legal liability directly or indirectly caused by or contributed or arising from nuclear weapons.

How to Effect Insurance

- Proposal Form
- Veterinary Health Certificate from a qualified Veterinarian

- ❐ All birds in the farm should be covered.
- ❐ Farm should follow standard package of practices, vaccination schedule, deworming, and debeaking.
- ❐ Farm should maintain essential records as per insurer's specifications.

Claim Procedure

- ❐ In the event of death of birds immediate intimation should be given to the Company and the Insurer should be supplied with the following documents and required information :
  - Duly filled in claim form.
  - Vet. P.M. Report for sample birds.
  - Daily records of mortality, feeding etc.
  - Purchase invoices for the birds.
  - Any other point to substantiate the loss like photographs, medical bills, etc. as and when required.
- ❐ In case of alarming death/outbreak of epidemic nature immediate notice within 12 hours should be given to the Company and all birds should be segregated and produced to the representative of the Company or to any person authorised by the Company for inspection.
- ❐ Daily mortality details should be sent to the Company on weekly basis failing which report will be treated as nil for that particular week.
- ❐ Delay in reporting of the claim should be avoided and if there is delay for more than three days the claim can be treated as non-standard.
- ❐ In case of doubtful claims/farms for which claim ratio is adverse, Technical Report from an expert may be insisted for settlement of claim.

During the outbreak of epidemic/natural calamities in the farm, insured has to arrange emergency sale of live birds in the presence of the representative of the insurance company in order to avert or minimise the loss. In case the insured realises the value less than the valuation table agreed upon for the corresponding week then the difference will be paid to the insured in addition to the cost of dead birds as per terms and conditions of the policy.

❐❐❐

Chapter 13

Record Keeping - Commercial Flocks

Data are kept for the purpose of performance analysis and financial appraisal during the process of brooding, growing and slaughtering of commercial turkeys. Daily inspection of production data allows the informed stockman to better manage his flock(s) and make effective responses to any changes or deviations from the expected norms.

1. Placement Data

- Number of day old poults.
- Strain and sex.
- Flock(s) names/codes.
- Date and time of arrival.
- Poult quality (size/uniformity etc.) and number of dead on arrivals (DOAs).
- House floor area.

2. Mortality

- Daily mortality (all breeder flocks together) - it is common to record natural deaths and culled mortality separately.
- Weekly and cumulative flock mortality (number and percentage).

3. Live Weight

- Weekly average live weight.
- Daily average live weight if automatic weighers are in use.

4. Egg Production

- Daily production.

5. Feed

- Date of delivery.
- Quantity delivered.
- Type (compound crumbs/pellet, whole grain).
- Ration name/codes.
- Feed quality (e.g. whether pellets are hard or break down to dust).
- Feed intake.

6. Water

- Daily consumption volume.
- Chlorination level and check dates and results.
- Environment.
- House temperature (daily maximum and minimum).
- External daily temperature.
- Air quality, e.g. dust, moisture levels and occasional measurement of ammonia.
- Daily litter quality (often a simple point score can be used e.g. 1 to 4, where 1 is very good, dry and friable and 4 is very poor, wet and dirty).
- Litter used - quantity/date of additional litter added (No. bags/ bales and weight of each unit).
- Weekly checks of standby generators.

7. Medication & Vaccination

- Date(s) administered.
- Whether routine or not (part of Veterinary Health Plan or following Veterinary Prescription).
- Type (name and batch numbers).
- Amounts used & method of administration.

8. Miscellaneous

- Rodent control record.
- Cleaning out dates.
- Detergents, disinfectants and fumigant used.
- Hygiene checks (total bacterial counts).
- Weekly checks of standby generators.

Turkey farm records

1. Breeder Flock : Daily register

Variety of turkey : .... Number birds housed : ....

Pen No : .... Date of hatch : ....

Date of housing : ....

Month	January			February			March		
Date	Mortality (No.)	Eggs (No.)	Feed issued kg	Mortality (No.)	Egg (No.)	Feed issued kg	Mortality (No.)	Egg (No.)	Feed issued kg
1									
2									
3									
.									
.									
.									
.									
.									
.									
.									
30									

2. Turkey poults : Daily register

Name of the farm and address : ....
Date of hatch : ....
Name of the variety : ....
No. of turkey poults housed initially : ....
Average body weight : ....
Pen no. : ....

Date	Age in days	Mortaility (No.)	Feed Intake /day (kg)	Feed Intake /week (kg)	Average body weight in (grams)	Feed conversion ratio

3. Vaccination schedule

Date	Vaccine	Date of manufacture of vaccine	Expiry date of vaccine	Quantity of vaccine given

4. Sales register

No. of turkey poults : ....
Variety of turkey sold : ....
Total live body weight : ....
Average body weight : ....

Date	No. of turkeys sold	Total body weight (Kg)	Average body weight (kg)	Price / kg

□□□

Chapter 14

Hatchery Management

Incubation

The incubation period in turkey is 28 days. There are two methods of incubation.

Natural Incubation with Broody Hens

Turkeys are good brooders naturally and the broody hen can hatch 10-15 numbers of eggs.

Artificial Incubation

In artificial incubation, eggs are hatched with the help of incubators. The measure of success of any hatchery is the number of first-quality chicks produced. This number is expressed as a percentage of all eggs set for incubation and is normally termed hatchability. Only clean eggs with good eggshell and shape should be placed for hatching to get 60-80% hatchability and healthy poults.

Physical Requisites of Incubation

- Temperature
- Relative humidity
- Ventilation
- Position and Turning of eggs

Types of Incubators

There are two types of incubators

- Still air incubators, which have no air circulating within the incubator.
- Forced draft incubators, in which air circulates for a more even temperature throughout the incubator.

Care of Hatching Eggs

Proper egg care is important to achieve maximum hatchability and produce healthy, vigorous chicks. Ideal practices in collecting, handling, cooling, storing and transporting of hatching eggs must be practiced.

Nests

Nests are to be kept clean. Clean and fresh nesting material is to be provided. During the first few weeks, birds tend to scratch the material out of the nests. Extra attention has to be given to replace the nest material early in the laying period. Droppings, broken eggs and soiled material are to be removed from nest promptly and replaced with clean fresh nest material.

Collection

Eggs are to be collected frequently, 4 times a day and more often during extremes of hot or cold weather. Hands are to be frequently washed when handling eggs.

Selection of Hatching Eggs

Select clean, nest-laid eggs for hatching purposes. All floor, slat and dirty eggs are to be gathered and kept separate from hatching eggs and utilized as market eggs only. If eggs are soiled, it is preferable to clean them with sandpaper and egg brush. Select hatching eggs that are uniform in size (minimum recommended weight 70 g for meat-type), shape and colour, with good sound shells. Do not set malformed, porous-shelled, doubled-yolked eggs or eggs with cracks.

Hatching Egg Sanitation

The goal of any breeder operation is to provide clean eggs to the hatchery. Sanitation is important in every step of collection, handling and storage.

Fumigation

Fumigation with formaldehyde gas has been an effective method of sanitation of hatching egg. The formaldehyde provides excellent bacterialcide on contact and it is very easy to fumigate a large number of eggs at a time.

Fumigation materials per 100 cubic feet

Concentration	Formaldehyde	Potassium permanganate
Single strength	40 cc	20 grams
Double strength	80 cc	40 grams
Triple strength	120 cc	60 grams

Fumigation procedures

Eggs are placed in an air tight cabinet or room immediately after collecting the eggs. Close all the vents. Place the recommended amount of fumigation materials in the bottom of the cabinet or in the room. Close the door and fumigate the cabinet or room for 30 minutes. Open the vents and turn on the exhaust fan; then open the door to remove fumes. Remove the eggs to the holding room.

Egg Storage

Eggs are to be stored at 14–15°C (57-59°F). The humidity in the egg store is to be kept between 70–80% RH. Eggs are routinely stored before incubation for between 2 to 7 days with minimal impact on hatching success. Incubating eggs on the day that they are laid or, to a lesser extent, after one day of storage can depress hatchability. Extending egg storage beyond 7 days will result in lower hatchability, the longer the storage the greater the effect. The age of a breeder flock affects the ability of eggs to withstand long egg storage.

Candling

The candling of hatching eggs is done to determine fertility. It is also useful in determining other sources of breeder flock or hatchery failures, such as percentages of eggs set upside down, cracked and embryos that have died early. Many hatcheries incorporate the candling procedure into their quality control program to monitor the week-to-week status of their breeders throughout the life of the flocks. Candling can be done as early as five days of incubation, but errors in candling often occur at this time. Due to the rapid growth rate of the embryos during the second week of incubation, very few candling errors are made after 14th day of incubation. Clear eggs consist of infertiles and eggs with early dead embryos emit more light than eggs with viable embryos. Clear eggs are removed from the tray to be broken out. Candling with a spot candler is a little slower, but it is more accurate.

Commercial Incubation

Multi-Stage Incubation Procedure

Multi-stage incubation is where the machines are operated continuously, with eggs being set and transferred in the machine. Multi-stage incubation uses the heat generated by the eggs at the end of incubation to warm the eggs at the start of incubation. The alternative system is single-stage incubation where all the eggs within the incubator are at the same stage of development. The temperature and relative humidity in setter and hatcher are as follows:

	Temperature (°C)	Relative humidity (%)
Setter	37.5	61 - 63
Hatcher	37	85 - 90

Setter Management

Setting Eggs

To avoid temperature shock to the embryo and consequent condensation on the shell, eggs should be removed from the egg storage room and brought to room temperature (24-27°C).

Setting Patterns

Multi-stage incubators rely on the efficient transfer of heat from the eggs at the end of incubation to those at the start of incubation. Eggs are normally set within a multi-stage machine either weekly or twice weekly.

Egg Transfer

Eggs are removed from the setter after 24 or 25 days and transferred to the hatcher trays. This is done for two reasons. The eggs are laid on their sides to allow free movement of the chick out of the shell at hatching. It also assists hygiene; large quantities of fluff are generated during hatching and spread this potential contamination around the hatchery. Transferring too early or too late will result in embryos being subjected to sub-optimal conditions causing lower hatchability.

Operations of Hatcher

Most hatcheries hatch twice a week from each hatcher. The hatcher will be washed and disinfected between hatches, which means durability of construction and ease of cleaning are vital factors. Air supply to the hatchers should be 15 cfm/1000 eggs (0.42 m /minute/ 1000 eggs). From point of transfer to pipping, airflow and humidity in the hatcher has to be maintained the same as in the setter. Moisture is important during the hatching process to ensure the shell membranes remain soft and pliable so that the chick can escape unhindered. When pipping starts, the moisture level will rise causing the wet bulb temperature to also rise. At this point, the vent will require adjustment to maintain this level. A few hours before take off the vent is opened to increase air supply for the chicks. Hatcher temperatures are usually slightly lower than those of the setter to reduce the risk of overheating.

Hatching Phase

The hatching phase is when the poults start to pip all the way around the eggshell and hatch from the egg. In a hatcher that contains eggs that are from one breeder flock and have not been stored for a long period, this phase will typically take 36 hours between the first and last poult hatching. As poults start to hatch they are wet and release a lot of water vapour into the hatcher, resulting in a rise in humidity. Once the natural rise in humidity starts most hatcheries increase the hatcher humidity setting for the rest of the hatching phase to match the natural rise in humidity. However, there is little scientific evidence that this is necessary and it is likely the main benefit is preventing a high humidity alarm. Ventilation should never be restricted in hatchers where the principle method of cooling the machine is by using air.

Drying Phase

Once the last poult has hatched the humidity in the hatcher is decreased and the ventilation increased so that the poults dry. Typically 6 hours should be sufficient for drying the poults, do not over extend the drying period as it will result in dehydrated poults. Once the hatch has finished and the poults are dry then it is best to remove the poults from the hatcher and hold them in poult boxes.

Chick Pull Out and Processing

Chicks are ready to be taken off when most of them are dry and fluffed up, with a few (about 5%) still having some moisture on the backs of their necks. A common mistake is to allow chicks to spend too long in the hatchers so they dehydrate excessively. Dehydration of chicks may result from incorrect adjustment of setting time for egg age or excessive weight loss during incubation. Similarly, if they are "green" (i.e. not yet ready) check setting times and also check for opportunities for the eggs to have become cooled down in incubation, reducing the rate of development. Upon pulling chicks, they have to be separated from their debris, graded into first quality and culls, and counted into boxes. Some hatcheries carry out addtional operations such as :

- Sexing, primarily using feather-sexing with broilers but also vent sexing with breeding stock.
- Vaccination, sprayed or injected, using hand or automatic vaccinators.
- Beak trimming.

Chick Dispatch Boxes

Chick dispatch boxes are usually made to hold 12, 25, 50 or 100 day-old chicks, plus a small percentage of replacements. There are many patterns on the market, each with their own arrangement of air holes to permit safe transport of the chicks under any given set of climatic conditions likely to be encountered in this country.

Sending Out Day-Old Chicks

Chicks reach their destination by lorry, by rail or their new buyers may collect them at the hatchery. Chicks are to be culled at the time the boxes are being filled and only those that attain a satisfactory standard should be sent out. The points that should be shown by sound chicks are:

- *Health and vigour*: indicated by round, bright eyes, sturdy legs, ability to stand firmly, and a well grown fluffy down.
- *Good size*: this will of course vary somewhat with type, breed and egg size.
- *Trueness to type*: any obvious anomalies such as incorrect colouring or comb type should be rejected.
- *Freedom from deformity*: any chick with crooked legs or toes, odd shaped beaks, eyes missing or stuck up, pasty vents or unhealed navels should be discarded.

□□□

Chapter 15

Preparation of Compound Feeds - Present Status

Domestic animals continue to make important contributions to global food supply and, as a result, animal feeds have become an increasingly critical component of the integrated food chain. Livestock products account for about 30 percent of the global value of agriculture and 19 percent of the value of food production, and provide 34 percent of protein and 16 percent of the energy consumed in human diets. Meeting consumer demand for more meat, milk, eggs and other livestock products is dependent to a major extent on the availability of regular supplies of appropriate, cost-effective and safe animal feeds.

Compound Feed Sector

The world's manufactured tonnage exceeds 560 million tons. In India; 58 billion eggs, 2.7 million broilers and 112 million tonnes of milk are produced annually. The present demand for the total compound feed in India is estimated at 68 million tons and is expected to increase to 74 million tons by 2012.

The principal cost in the manufacture of compound feeds is that of raw materials; this may amount to as much as 80 percent, or more, of the manufacturing costs in large size mills. Due to increasing transportation costs and the need to conserve foreign exchange, the tendency in most developing countries is to use locally available ingredients. Traditionally, the animal feed milling industry has been linked to the supply of raw materials. In recent years, due to increasing world demand, most feed ingredients have become articles of international commerce. As a result, quality has become more consistent for most feedstuffs. Availability is often just a matter of agreeing upon prices between trading partners. Feed mills, too, are now being located in areas where they can take best advantage of markets for finished products and of alternate supply sources for raw materials.

Feed manufacturing has not been firmly established as an entrepreneurial avenue in Tamilnadu. To improve the productivity and profit in poultry industry, entrepreneurs can come forward to start a small or large scale feed manufacturing unit. In feed manufacturing the quality of feed ingredients obtained and cost plays a major role in determining the profitability of the sector. In the past ten years there has not been much change in the energy rich feed ingredients used. But among the protein supplements, groundnut oil cake has been replaced either partly or fully by soyabean meal.

The major reasons for indecision in starting a feed manufacturing enterprise include:

- Quality problems encountered while obtaining feed ingredients
- Difficulties faced in procurement of feed milling equipments

There is a common misconception among the farmers that, to start a feed manufacturing enterprise the initial investment is very high. But, there are equipments which are available for small scale production. The selection of equipment can be done according to the requirement. Pulverisers of 1.5 hp are available which can grind upto 300 kg of feed per day. To grind 1000 kg of feed per day, medium sized equipment like hammer mill can be used. To grind about 5 to 10 tonnes of feed per day automated feed units can be installed. The cost of feed mill equipment ranges from Rs.25, 000/- to Rs.10, 00,000/- and above; based on the capacity. The profit obtained in poultry rearing can be increased substantially by providing them with quality feed. The entrepreneurs interested in starting feed manufacturing unit can obtain a decent profit by establishing it in a small or large scale.

Chapter 16

Nutrients in Feed

Feed is required for growth, maintenance and reproductive process of the body. The feed given to poultry consists chiefly of cereals and by-products of plant and animal origin. These feed contain substances known as nutrients. There are more than 40 nutrients required by poultry. They are arranged into six groups according to their chemical nature and functions they perform.

- Water
- Carbohydrates
- Proteins
- Fats
- Vitamins
- Minerals

Water

Some water is available in the feed itself (metabolic water), but the bulk of it has to be provided separately. Water is required for various body functions. The water content of the body of an adult turkey is about 60 to 65%and an egg contains two- thirds water. When drinking water is not provided for a day to the layers there may be a complete cessation of egg production. Poultry can survive for a long time without taking any solid food but very quickly suffers if there is a shortage of water. Hence, an ample supply of water has to be provided to the birds. For every kg of feed, 2-3 kg of water is consumed. Water intake at 33.3°C in hot tropics is 50 per cent higher or double than at 21.1°C in the temperate regions. The water has to be at the right temperature. The best temperature is 10-11 0 C but this is not practically attainable in the tropics. The water has to be free from excessive salts which might have a laxative effect. Potable water has to be provided and it has to be constantly kept free from droppings and litter material.

Carbohydrates

Carbohydrates are the main source of energy for the birds. Energy is not a nutrient by itself, but a property that a nutrient possesses. Turkey needs energy for body maintenance, movement, growth and for the production of eggs and meat. Carbohydrates are available in plenty in plant sources. These are classified as a) solubie carbohydrates: they have more energy, are easily digested and consist mostly of starches, sugars and pentosans b) crude fibre: it has low energy, it is not easily digested and consists mostly of cellulose, lignin, hemicellulose, etc.The feed given to the turkeys contain about 60 to 65 % of energy rich supplements. The factors affecting energy requirement are environmental temperature, diseases and feed intake. The feed intake in turn varies with the size, level of egg production and health status of the bird. The density of feed and physical form also affects the feed intake.

Protein

It is essential for both growth as well as production. The proteins in the body of the bird or in the eggs are made from the amino acids assembled in the gut in the process of digestion and then modified in other organs. It is therefore necessary that these ingredients have to come from feeds which have similar combination of amino acid. Protein nutrition, therefore, consists in identifying the amino acid requirements of the turkeys and then supplying these directly (essential amino acids) (arginine, cystine, histidine, isoleucine, leucine, lysine, methionine and phenyl alanine) or supplying in feedstuffs which will be broken down into simpler nitrogenous compounds from which, in turn, the animal's amino acid requirement can be synthesized. (non-essential amino acids) (alanine, aspartine, glycine, hydroxyproline, proline and serine).

Concept of Balance of Amino Acids

An excess or deficiency of one amino acid upset the amino acid balance and the usefulness of the entire feed. It is therefore, necessary to formulate rations to achieve an appropriate balance of amino acids avoiding both deficiencies and also surpluses.

Idea of Limiting Amino Acid

It is a matter of identifying economic responses of amino acids and trying to satisfy them. A nutritionist has to take note of those amino acids of which a decrease in input causes a bigger decrease in performance than a similar unit decrease with the inclusion of others. These are known as limiting amino acids and one tries to identify them in sequence as first limiting, second limiting and so on. Methionine and lysine as first limiting and second limiting acids respectively. The order of amino acid limitation in a feed will be influenced by the ingredients used. Thus where soya-bean meal supplies the bulk of the protein the first limiting amino acid will usually be methionine. On the other hand, where cottonseed meal provides the protein, lysine is likely to be first limiting.

Synthetic Amino Acids

Methionine and lysine are available as separate manufactured ingredients at an economical cost.

Variations in Protein Requirement

The amount of protein required by turkeys varies considerably according to age and stage of production. The demand for protein during the first six to eight weeks of life,during egg production and the moult are extremely high. Also, protein requirements are closely associated with the energy level of the total diet- the higher the energy level, the greater the percentage of protein that is required.

Fat

Fats and oils are the group of nutrients which help to supply the turkey with energy. They are always of vegetable or animal origin. Compared with carbohydrate, weight for weight, one part of fat yields 2.25 times more energy. Fat can be included to a rate of 5-10%, which helps in increasing the palatability of the feed and also utilization of fat soluble vitamins. Additionally; unsaturated fatty acids, linoleic, linolenic and arachidonic are considered as essential nutrients for poultry. But inclusion of higher amount fat is not advisable because it will increase the feed cost and also increase the occurrence of rancidity.

Vitamins

Vitamins are organic substances needed by the body in minimum amounts for normal growth, health and production. Vitamins are grouped into two classes on the basis of their solubility: fat- soluble and water-soluble. Vitamins are organic compounds not synthesized in the body tissues and are required in very small amounts in diet. They are not structural components of the body but rather they most commonly function as co-enzymes or regulators of metabolism. The thirteen vitamins required by poultry are partly the fat- soluble ones; namely vitamin A, D, E and K; and water- soluble ones, namely thiamine, riboflavin, nicotinic acid, folic acid, biotin, pantothenic acid, pyridoxine, B12 and Choline.

Mineral salts

Minerals are required for skeletal tissue development and maintenance. They form 10% of the total weight of eggs and 3 to 5% of a turkey's body weight. Calcium, phosphorus and magnesium account for 25%, 12% and 0.5% respectively of the bone. Calcium is 40% of egg shell, 98% of which is CaCo3. The major minerals are calcium, phosphorus, sodium, potassium, magnesium and chlorine. The trace elements needed by the turkey are iron, manganese, copper, molybdenum, zinc and selenium. Those that are likely to be adequate are potassium, magnesium, zinc, silicon and fluorine, while the likely deficient ones are calcium, phosphorus, sodium, chlorine, manganese, iodine, iron, copper and cobalt.

□□□

Chapter 17

Classes of Feeds

Classes of Feeds by Composition and Usage

Feeds are grouped into eight classes on the basis of their composition in the way they are used for formulating diets.

Classes of Feeds by Composition and Usage

Code	Class Description*	
1	Dry forages and roughages	Hay; straw; fodder (aerial part); stover (aerial part without ears, without husks or aerial part without heads); other products with more than 18 percent crude fibre (dry basis); hulls. This class includes all forages and roughages cut and cured. Forages or roughages are low in net energy per unit weight, usually because of the high fibre content. Thus, such products as seed coats, pods, rice bran, etc. are included in this group.

2	Pasture, range plants, and forages fed green	Included in this group are all forage feeds either not cut (including feeds cured on the stem) or cut and fed fresh.
3	Silages	This class includes only ensiled forages (maize, alfalfa, grass, etc.), but not ensiled fish, grain, roots and tubers.
4	Energy feeds	Included in this group are products with less than 20 percent protein (dry basis) and less than 18 percent crude fibre (dry basis) as, for example, fish, grain, mill by-products,
5	Protein supplements	This class includes products which contain 20 percent or more of protein (dry basis) from animal origin (including ensiled products) as well as oil meals, gluten, etc.
6	Mineral supplements	
7	Vitamin supplements (including ensiled yeast)	
8	Additives	This class includes further feed supplements as antibiotics, colouring materials, flavours, hormones and medicants.

* Short feed names are used with or without the genus, species or variety

Energy Feeds

According to the notation in the outline classification, energy feeds are low-protein concentrates. The upper limit for protein is conveniently set at 20 percent, because this figure then includes wheat bran which is otherwise difficult to classify. However, it is the entire seed of the cereals that is the typical energy feed.

Chemical Characteristics

Protein

An energy feed is likely to contain about 12 percent crude protein of which between 75 and 80 percent is digestible. All feeds of this group show lysine as their first limiting amino acid, which is of importance in the choice of a protein supplement to be used in a balanced ration. It also explains why substitution between energy feeds is not likely to alter appreciably the protein quality of the mixture.

Typical Composition of Cereal Grains

Feed Name	Crude Protein		Ether extract	Carbohydrate	
	Total (%)	Chemical score	(%)	Crude fibre (%)	N-free extract (%)
Barley, grain	11.6	20	1.9	5.0	68.2
Corn, grain	9.3	28	4.3	2.0	71.2
Oats, grain	11.8	464	4.5	11.0	58.5
Rye, grain	11.9	50	1.6	2.0	71.8
Sorghum, milo, grain	11.0	-	2.8	2.0	71.6
Wheat grain	12.7	37	1.7	3.0	70.0
Average	11.4	-	2.8	4.2	6.8

Ash

Energy feeds are low in calcium. In practice, they are often neglected in making calculations for calcium supplementation. The content of phosphorus, on the other hand, is enough.

Carbohydrates

About two thirds of the weight of the seed is likely to be starch, which will usually be about 95 percent digested. Not only is this high concentration of easily digested carbohydrate the distinguishing feature of energy feeds, but variation in this characteristic determines the consequences of substituting among feeds of this category.

Fat

The cereal grains belonging to the energy feeds normally contain from 2 to 5 percent ether extract, but a few by-product feedstuffs contain up to 13 percent fat, as does rice feed, the mill-run by-products of the manufacture of polished rice. The-fat of non-oily seeds is concentrated in the germ, and any processing that removed an appreciable proportion of the protein or carbohydrate, but not of the germ will leave a by-product with higher fat content than the parent seed.

Crude Fibre

The average crude fibre of the energy feeds is about 6 percent but individual feeds vary considerably. The upper limit for concentrates is taken as 18 percent, In particular, the coarse grain (barley and oats) may show wide deviations in fibre from sample to sample, ordinarily because of either an increase in hull or a decrease in the starch filling of the groat. Differences in fibre affect markedly their available energy value and hence their relative feeding value. The most important consequence of substitution between energy feeds is usually traceable to differences in the crude fibre of the products. Fibres of different origin are often quite different nutritionally. It is also generally true that amount of fibre and of available energy of energy feeds of feed mixtures are negatively correlated. Thus, raising the percentage of fibre means greater bulkiness and lower available energy, which in turn demand larger amounts of feed. In other words, high-fibre feeds are relatively less efficient sources of productive energy.

Non-Chemical Characteristics of Energy Feeds

Bulk

In a general consideration of characteristics of energy feeds as a group, there are some non-chemical characteristics we should mention. The first one in order of importance is probably bulkiness. A bulky feed is relatively low in its yield of biologically available energy.

Relationship of Bulk Density, and Percent of Fibre Energy Feeds

Feed	Bulk density (g/litre)	Percent of fibre
Wheat, grain	810	4
Corn, grain	750	2
Rye, grain	750	2
Barley, grain	560	6
Oats, grain	355	10
Wheat, standard middlings	385	7
Wheat, bran	255	9
Oat, mill feed	150	27

Quality in Energy Feeds

Sample-to-sample variation in quality is a special problem with energy feeds. The important feeds of this group fall into two subgroups of crude fibre. Corn, wheat, and rye or a type of plant seed that is without an enveloping hull make up one group. Barley and oat kernels, on the other hand, after threshing, remain encased in their flowering glumes, and because of this attribute, they are referred to as coarse grains.

Maize / Corn

Of the energy feeds of the low-fibre group, maize is the key feed in livestock rations. As seen in Table it is the lowest in crude protein and highest in available energy. Maize contains around 9% crude protein and 3370 kcal energy. This can be included upto 60% in turkey feed. Maize provides yellow colouration to the egg yolk, the leg of the turkeys and also its nostrils and skin. The precursors of vitamin A like carotene and xanthophylls are rich in maize.

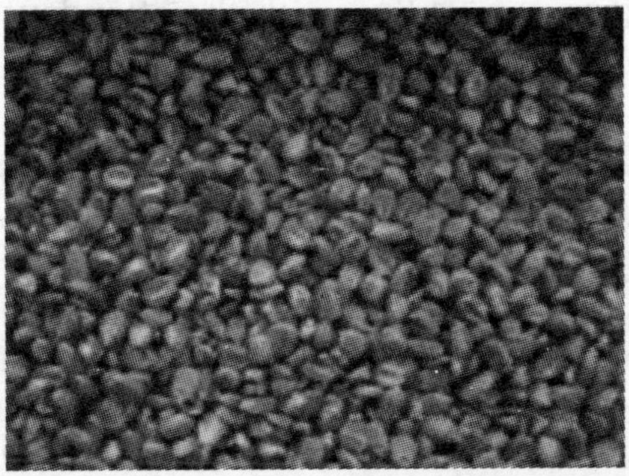

Relative Values of Energy Feeds as Carbohydrate Concentrates

Grain	Percent of protein (Morrison)	Percent of net energy (Morrison)
Corn (maize), grain	74	100
Barley, grain	91	86
Kafir, grain	92	93
Milo, grain	87	93
Oats, grain	92	88
Rye, grain	74	86
Wheat, grain	100	97

Corn, like all other grains, is subject to variation in make-up because of varietal differences and the specific conditions under which it is grown and harvested. Locally produced samples may differ from published average figures for chemical composition.

Economically the variation in the protein percentage of corn may be highly important. In compounding batches of balanced rations, much more protein supplement may be needed with low-protein corn than with high-protein corn to prepare a mixture of some desired percentage of protein

Two other characteristics of corn should be mentioned. The one concerns its fat (or ether extract) content, which is higher than the average of energy feeds. This is both an asset and a liability. There is little doubt that a part of the acceptability of corn to animals is traceable to its fat component, not on the physical nature of the ground grain. The high fat level, however, can be a distinct liability, since ground corn goes rancid easily. The effect may be slight, and may represent merely a superficial loss of palatability, or it may be extensive enough to result in heating or molding with the attendant loss in nutritive value. In general, ground corn cannot be stored without risk of such damage.

The other characteristic of corn is its moisture content. Samples of corn as harvested are likely to vary more in water content than those of any other grain. They may range from 8 percent water for fully mature corn to 35 percent for frosted immature grain. Ear corn containing over 25 percent water, and shelled corn containing more than about 15 percent, will not store without damage in the usual types of cribs or bins. Aside from the effect of moisture content on storage, the nutritive value of the grain will decline as it is "diluted" with more and more water.

Wheat

Wheat contains about 11% crude protein, and 3090 kcal energy. This can be included up to 50% in the diet of turkeys.

Rice

Since it is much used in human diet, inclusion of rice in turkey feed is generally avoided. It contains about 8% crude protein and 2670 kcal of energy. Broken rice can be included in the turkey feeds.

Millets

Ragi, jowar, bajra are the commonly available millets. These can be included in the feed as such or in broken farm. These contains about 3.5-12% crude protein and 2950 kcal of energy. Millet can be included up to the rate of 10-20% in the diet.

White Sorghum

This contains about 10% crude protein and 3260 k cal energy. This can be included upto 25% in the feed of turkey poults and 40% in adult turkey feed.

Red Sorghum

This contains about 11% crude protein and 3090 k cal energy. This can be included upto 10% in the feed of turkey poults and 20% in adult turkey feed. This contains the anti nutritional factor called tannin. If the feed contains a higher level of tannin, it may cause a reduction in the egg production.

Coarse Grains

As already implied, it is the glume on the hull that accounts for the higher fibre of the so-called coarse grains.

The difficulty with these grains is that the proportions of groat to hulls are widely variable within the species, and are further modified by seasonal growing conditions. Not only do the seeds themselves vary but the crops as harvested include, in addition to the grain intentionally planted, the seeds from an assortment of other plants of volunteer origin from a previous crop or from weed impurities in the planting grain. Corn (maize) and wheat are relatively free (or are easily freed) from such contaminants, but with barley and oats purity of sample is often a factor influencing feeding value.

Cereal by-products

Rice Bran with Germ

Rice bran with germ is primarily the pericarp or bran layer and the germ portions of the rice kernel. The crude protein level is approximately 13.3 percent; crude fat, 15.0 percent; and crude fibre, 11.0 percent.

Deoiled Rice Bran

This contains about 14% crude protein and 2,240 kcal energy. The crude fiber content is 21%. This can be included in the turkey feed up to 20-40%.

Rice Polishing

Rice polishing is the outer portions of the rice kernel produced by the process used in producing polished white rice. Rice polishing has a crude protein level of 11.8 percent; crude fat, 13.2 percent; and crude fibre, 3.0 percent.

Wheat Bran

Wheat bran is the coarse outer covering of the wheat berry. Sometimes screenings are ground and added to the bran. Wheat bran contributes bulk to feeds and is a source of carbohydrates, protein, minerals and vitamins. Generally, wheat bran will have a crude protein level of 14-17 percent; crude fat, 3-4.5 percent; and crude fibre, 10.5-12 percent.

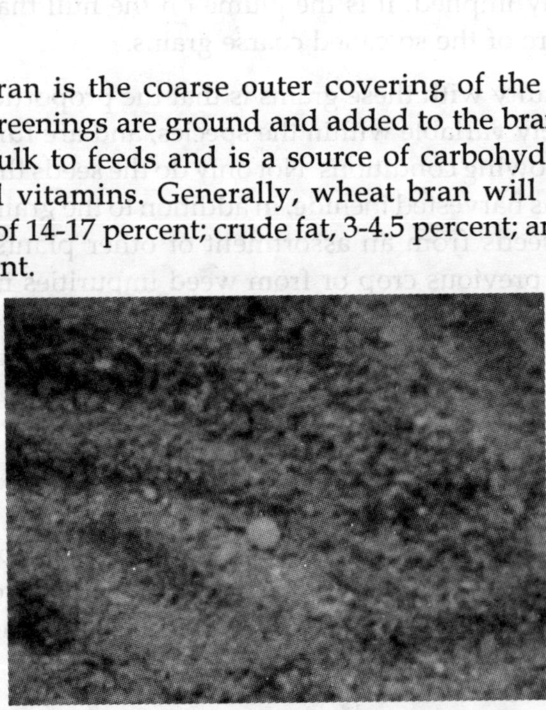

Protein Supplements

Products of Plant Origin

As indicated in the feed classification, the protein supplements of plant origin divide quite naturally into two subgroups - one containing the feeds with 20 to 30 percent total crude protein, the other those with 30 to 45 percent crude protein.

The chief difference between these two types of supplements is in protein content, the higher protein being associated with a lower carbohydrate analysis. The 20 to 30 percent group is made up primarily of by-products-of wet milling, brewing, or distilling of corn or barley. These by-products tend to be high in crude fibre. The feeds of the other group are almost entirely residues of oil bearing seeds, which have been processed by chemical extraction or by expression to remove most of the oil.

Chemical scores show that the feeds in the 20 to 30 percent range have poorer-quality protein than those in the higher-protein category. Perhaps the reason for this difference is that less of the germ proteins are removed by fat extraction than by water treatments involved in wet milling or brewing. The feeds of this lower-protein group are by-products either of corn or barley, and the chief, or at least the first, limiting factor in their quality is a deficiency of lysine. At the moment there is no experimental evidence of qualitative differences between these two proteins.

Solvent-Extracted Oilseed Residues

In spite of the over-all better quality, the first limiting amino acid of linseed and cottonseed is lysine, but with peanut meal the sulfur-containing amino acids, methionine and cystine, are relatively the more deficient, with lysine standing second, soybean proteins, on the other hand, are probably the most complete of any of the plant seed proteins.

Crude Fibre

The feeds belonging to the lower-protein category are likely to have higher crude fibre content than those of the oil meal group. The important factor here is the bulkiness of the feed. As a ration is made bulkier by the inclusion of light feeds, the quantity (by volume) of it required to yield the amount of digestible energy called for by the feeding standard increases rather rapidly.

Calcium and Phosphorus

In any case, these feeds will usually constitute not more than 20 percent of the final meal mixture fed and their calcium content, therefore, will not be important in changing the calcium content of the ration.

The problem of phosphorus, however, is somewhat different. This element in feeds is quite likely to be correlated with protein content. Thus, high-protein feeds commonly provide more phosphorus than low-protein feeds.

Fat

The fat content of oil-bearing seed by-products must be taken into account sometimes if they are to be used for certain classes of livestock. Most vegetable oils, if fed to meat animals in any appreciable amounts for a month or more previous to the slaughter of the animals, tend to produce soft, oily carcass fat. Thus the feeding of the oilseeds as grown on the farm is not ordinarily desirable. Extraction of the oil leaves a residue that may contain from almost none to 12 percent fat, depending on the process and the efficiency with which it is operating.

Expeller oil meals will contain about 8 percent fat. The use of solvent extraction is increasingly common, with the result that the fat content of oil meals so treated is reduced to about 1 percent. This reduction of fat means an increase in protein and in carbohydrate concentration, but a reduction of about 5 percent in energy value. The alteration of protein level is great enough to be nutritionally and economically important, but the changes in the other nutrients are not likely to have measurable effects in the final ration.

Soybean Meal

The special role of soybean meal as a protein supplement requires comment. Because of its higher biological value, this feed has now replaced most of the meat meal and fish meal, which were in the past the mainstay of protein quality in rations for non-herbivorous animals.

Considering the protein quality of soybean meal this leads to the conclusion that the chief advantage it has over linseed meal protein is its markedly greater concentration of lysine, the amino acid that is ordinarily the first deficiency in the energy feeds. This can be included upto 40% in turkey feed.

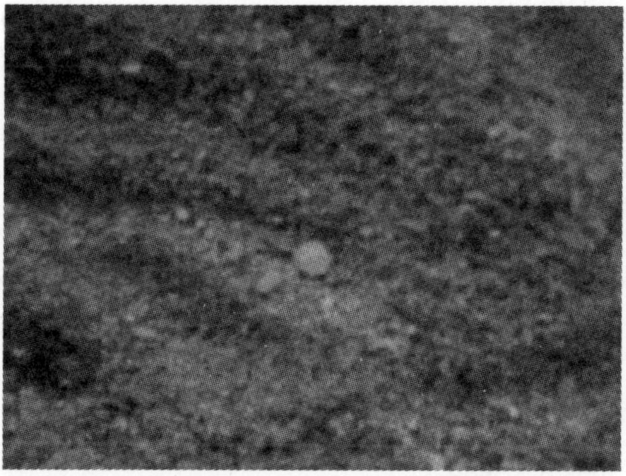

Soybean Meal Composition

Standard Definitions

Soybean Cake or Soybean Chips is the product after most of the oil is extracted from whole soybeans by pressure or solvents from soybeans. A name descriptive of the process of manufacture, such as "expeller', "hydraulic" or "solvent extracted" is used in the brand name. It shall be designed and sold according to its protein content.

Soybean Meal is ground soybean cake, ground soybean chips or ground soybean flakes. A name descriptive of the process of manufacture, such as "expeller', "hydraulic" or "solvent extracted" is used in the brand name. It shall be designed and sold according to its protein content.

Soybean Mill Feed is the by-product resulting from the manufacture of soybean flour or grits and is composed of soybean hulls and offal from the tail of the mill. A typical analysis is 13% crude protein, 32% crude fiber and 13% moisture.

Soybean Mill Run is the by-product resulting from the manufacture of dehulled soybean meal and is composed of soybean hulls and such bean meats that adhere to the hull in normal milling operations. A typical analysis is 11% crude protein, 35% crude fiber and 13% moisture.

Soybean Hulls are a by-product of soybean processing consisting primarily of the outer covering of the soybeans or seed coat. A typical analysis is 10-12% crude protein, 36-40% crude fiber and 9-13% moisture.

Standard Specifications

Soybean Flakes and 44% Protein Soybean Meal are produced by cracking, heating and flaking soybeans and reducing the oil content of the conditioned product by the use of hexane or homologous hydrocarbon solvents. The extracted flakes are cooked and marketed as such or ground into meal. Standard specifications are as follows.

Protein	minimum	44.0%
Fat	minimum	0.5%
Filter	maximum	7.0%
Moisture	maximum	12.0%

Soybean Flakes and High Protein or Solvent Extracted Soybean Meal are produced by cracking, heating and flaking dehulled soybeans and reducing the oil content of the conditioned flakes by the use of hexane or homologous hydrocarbon solvents. The extracted flakes are cooked and marketed as such or ground into meal. Standard specifications are as follows.

Protein	minimum	47.5-49%
Fat	minimum	0.5%
Filter	maximum	3.3-3.5%
Moisture	maximum	12.0%

Cottonseed Meals

Cottonseed meal is produced in three protein levels. Cottonseed meals are classified as low gossypol if they contain less than 0.04 percent free gossypol. Forty-one percent cottonseed meal has a crude protein level of 41 percent; crude fat, 2 percent; and crude fibre, 12 percent. Forty-eight percent cottonseed meal has a crude protein level of 48 percent; crude fat, 1 percent; and crude fibre, 8 percent. Although all three cottonseed meals are solvent extracted, the lower protein meals may contain some hulls.

Groundnut Oil Cake

Ground nut oil cake is available in three different forms:

- Ghanni
- Expeller
- Solvent extracted

Ground nut oil cake is obtained by grinding the cake, chips or flakes obtained by removal of most of the oil from groundnut kernels by a mechanical or solvent extraction process. Ground nut oil cake will have a crude protein level of about 46 percent; crude fat, 1-7 percent; and crude fibre, 10-13 percent. This oil cake can be included up to 20% in turkey feeds.

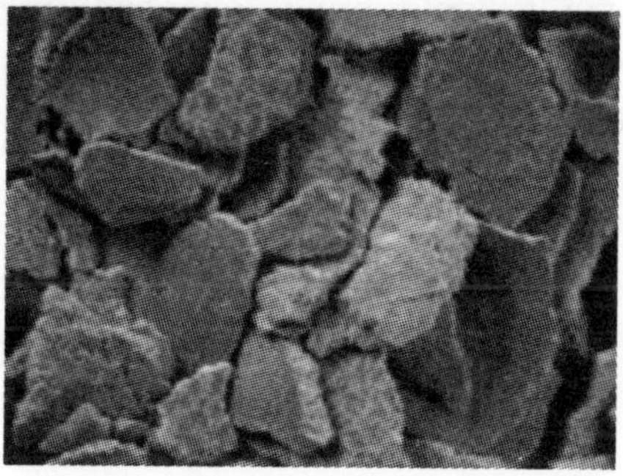

Sesame Oil Cake

Sesame oil cake from which oil is not extracted contains about 42% crude protein and 2,640 kcal of energy. The methionine content of sesame oil cake is much higher than other oil cakes. This can be included up to 5% in the diet. This is deficient in lysine and hence, this should be supplemented along with some animal protein supplements, so that the feed becomes balanced.

Sunflower Oil Cake

Solvent extracted sunflower oil cake contains about 27% crude protein and 1,900 kcal energy. This can be included up to 20% in adult turkey feed and upto 10% in turkey poult feed. Since the lysine content of this oil cake is much lesser, it should be supplemented along with certain animal protein supplements. This contains a higher level of pantothenic acid and niacin.

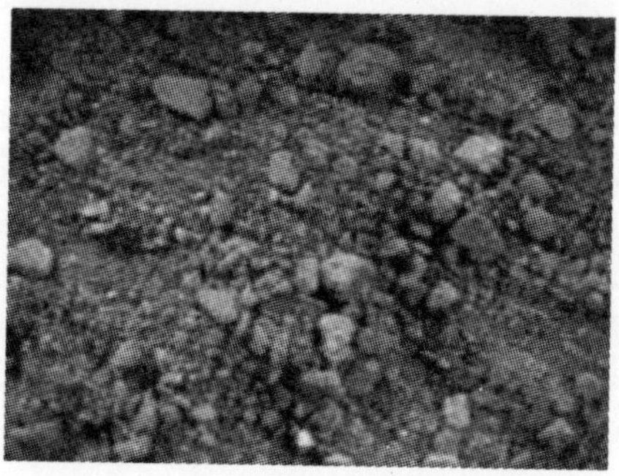

Protein Supplements of Animal and Marine Origin

Analogous to the high-protein feeds of plant origin is a group of edible by-products of animal or fish origin. These are usually employed to improve the total protein of energy feeds but, in addition, they contribute a mixture of amino acids quite different from that characteristic of most proteins of plant sources. For example, plant-seed proteins are usually seriously deficient in lysine. Meat, milk, and fish proteins, however, are relatively rich in this amino acid, though they are likely to be short of the sulfur-containing cystine and methionine.

The products belonging in this high-product group are more diverse in protein level than are feeds of any other protein category. The individual feeds frequently have unique properties affecting or limiting their use.

Composition of Typical Feeds of Animal or Marine Origin (All figures are percentages)

Feed	Protein Total	Digestible	Ether extract	Ash Ca	P	TDN
Meat meal	53	48	10	8.0	4.03	68
Meat and bone meal	51	45	10	11.0	5.07	65
Blood meal	80	62	2	0.3	0.22	61
Fish meal						
low ash (14)	71	66	6			78
high ash (31)	52	48	1			49
50% protein	53	49	4			55
70% protein	74	71	1			71
65% protein (oily)	68	65	10			87

It can be seen that the range of protein values is from 34 to 82 percent, which fat ranges from 1 to 15 percent, and that calcium and phosphorus for some of the feeds are present in supplementary amounts. There are several grades of fish meal, representing differences in processing which result in products of distinctly different characteristics as feeds. However, before dealing with individual products it should be noted that the general nutritional characteristic of the feeds of this group.

Protein Quality

There is a remarkable similarity in the amino-acid distribution of the different feeds. All carry as much or more lysine than is found in the protein of egg (which is usually taken as the standard of excellence for amino-acid assortment). As compared with the average cereal-grain protein, animal or marine proteins have a higher lysine level by about two and half times.

The isoleucine level of meat meal, fish meal is at least 50 percent higher than that in the mixed proteins of cereals, but blood meal is low in this amino acid. Because of their lysine and (in most cases) their isoleucine levels, the feeds of this group are valuable as supplements to the plant proteins, the combinations usually having a higher effective biological value than plant protein alone.

As a group, the feeds of this category are deficient in the sulfur-containing amino acids, cystine, and methionine. Methionine can, of course, be converted in vivo to cystine (although the reverse is not true). Hence, the combined deficiency of these two acids can be relieved by fortification of the diet with pure methionine, which is economically available as a feed supplement.

Ash

Another characteristic of this group of feeds is their high ash, especially their high calcium and phosphorus. Whereas the plant products contain less than 1 percent of either of these elements, and more often only 0.25 percent, meat and fish meals run from 5 to 11 percent calcium and from 3 to 5 percent phosphorus. These high levels are, of course, due to the presence of appreciable amounts of bone. In general, the higher the protein in either meat or fish meals, the lower the calcium and phosphorus. In many meal mixtures the desired supplementation of the energy feeds with these two minerals is accomplished by the use of meat or fish meals in amounts needed to adjust the protein quality or quantity.

Fat

Fish meals may have widely different fat percentages. Fat in either of these products is nutritionally a liability. It is unstable and, hence, complicates feed storage. The onset of rancidity not only may adversely affect palatability but may result in residues that catalyze the destruction of oxidizable nutrients in the ration, especially vitamins A and B.

Fish Meal

Fish meals are manufactured by cooking fish, pressing to remove water and oil, and then drying. Fish meals are often made from a single species of fish Thus, fish meal containing more than 9 percent fat is less desirable as a feed not only because of its oil, but because its high oil content is indicative of a product made from stale fish, or that is the result of bad processing. Fish meals that are residues of oil recovery by the "sun rotting" process are invariably oily, sometimes running as high as 20 percent ether extract. Such products should be avoided in the feeding of farm livestock. Since there is an upper limit to the desirable salt (NaCl) content of animal (especially poultry) rations, the salt content of fish meal is sometimes a factor limiting their usefulness. The maximum percentage of salt is 3 percent.

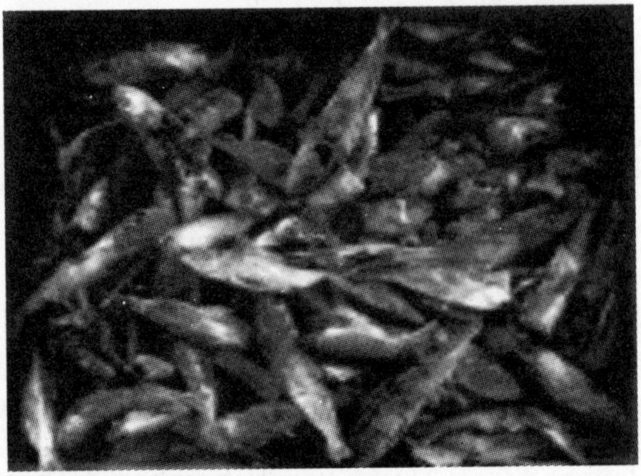

Meat and Bone Meal

Meat and bone meal is the dry rendered product derived from mammalian tissue, exclusive of hair, hoof, horn, manure and paunch contents. The relatively high fat content of meat and bone meal apparently helps protect the lysine content during rendering. Meat and bone meal generally contain a crude protein of 50 percent; fat, 8-11 percent; crude fibre 3 percent; phosphorus 4.4-5 percent; calcium, 8.8-10 percent; and ash about 30 percent.

Blood Meal

Blood meal is produced from clean fresh animal blood, exclusive of all extraneous material such as hair, stomach contents, etc. Blood meal may be dried by several processes, but most often by spray drying.

Spray dried blood meal has approximately a crude protein level of 85 percent; crude fat 0.5 - 3 percent; crude fibre 2.5 percent; ash 6 percent; and lysine, 9 - 11 percent, with an availability of 80-90 percent.

Vitamin and Mineral Supplements

Vitamins

Units of Potency

The presence in edible materials of nutrient substances needed for the survival and continued health of animals was discovered long before their chemical nature was learned. They were given the general name vitamins and the different vitamins were identified by letters, such as vitamin A or C. The potency of a foodstuff in any one of the first few vitamins discovered was originally expressed in terms of units. Later, in order that different research workers correlate their findings, international reference standards for certain vitamins were agreed upon. One could then measure vitamin potency of foods and express the daily need of animals in terms of these units.

Today, the needs of animals and the potency of foodstuff in a vitamin are usually expressed in terms of weight (milligrammes or microgrammes), though units of potency is still a common term in referring to vitamins A and D, and also occasionally in referring to B1 and B2. It desirable, therefore, to define at the outset the international standards and international units of potency (IU) for some of these vitamins.

Vitamin A. The international standard for vitamin A is pure crystalline vitamin A acetate. One international unit (IU) of vitamin A is 0.344 microgrammes of vitamin A acetate, which is equivalent to 0.3 microgrammes of vitamin A alcohol. It is distributed in capsules, each capsule containing 2 500 IU of vitamin A.

Provitamin A or carotene. The international standard for carotene is a sample of pure beta-carotene. One international unit of vitamin A is equivalent to 0.6 microgramme of beta-carotene; i.e., 1 mg of beta-carotene = 1 667 IU of vitamin A. International standards for vitamin A are based on the utilization by the rat of vitamin A and/or beta-carotene. Because other species do not convert carotene to vitamin A in the same ratio as rats, it is suggested that the conversion rates listed in Table can be used.

Conversion of Beta Carotene to Vitamin A for Different Species*

Species	Conversion of mg beta-carotene to IU vitamin A	Percent IU vitamin A activity (calculated from carotene)
Standard	1 = 1 667	100.0
Beef cattle	1 = 400	24.0
Dairy cattle	1 = 400	24.0
Sheep	1 = 400 -500	24.0 -30.0
Swine	1 = 500	30.0
Horses		
Growth	1 = 555	33.3
Pregnancy	1 = 333	20.0
Poultry	1 = 1 667	100.0
Dogs	1 = 833	50.0
Rat	1 = 1 667	100.0
Foxes	1 = 278	16.7
Cat	Carotene not utilized	
Mink	Carotene not utilized	
Man	1 = 556	33.0

*From: W.M. Beeson, Relative Potencies of Vitamin A and - Carotene for Animals. Federation Proc., XXIV (1965); p.924

Vitamin B_1. The international standard for vitamin B1 is pure synthetic thiamin hydrochloride. The IU is the potency of 3 microgramme of thiamin hydrochloride.

Vitamin B_2. This is pure riboflavin, and requirements are usually expressed as microgrammes per day. If expressed in Bourquin-Sherman units, 400 000 units = 1 g riboflavin.

Vitamin D. The international standard for vitamin D is pure crystalline irradiated 7-dehydrocholesterol (vitamin D3). One IU is 0.025 microgramme of the international standard. The USP reference standard is a solution of the international standard containing 400 IU in each g of solution.

Data on Vitamins Frequently Added to Rations

Name	Functions; units of potency, etc.	Good natural sources	Other sources (synthetic concentrates)	Supplementary amounts normally added/ ton meal, mixture*
Vitamin A (animal form) Carotene (plant form)	Stimulates formulation and development of body cells; a growth vitamin. Involved in dim-light vision. 0.6 micro-gramme carotene = 1 IU of vitamin A.	Leafy forage, fresh or preserved against oxidative loss. Milk or fish fat (variable). Yellow corn.	Pure crystalline vitamin A acetate, 3 000 000 IU/g. Mixed carotene 1000 000 IU/g.	1000000 IU
Vitamin D (D_2 is plant form; D_3 is animal form)	Faciliates absorption of calcium; related to normal bone formation. Irradiation by direct sun effectively supplies animals needed vitamin D. Poultry do not utilize D_2	Sun-cured, leafy hay to r animals (but not poultry).	Fortified fish oils, irradiated sterols for both poultry and animals. Crystalline D_2 or D_3 4000000 IU/g.	200000 IU
Riboflavin	Part of enzyme necessary for oxidation process in all living cells. Synthesized by micro-organisms in herbivora.	Liquid, condensed or dry milks. Dried leafy forage. Distillery soluble. Dried brewers' yeast.	Pure synthetic riboflavin, 400 000 BS units/g 1 g has potency of 100 lb skim milk powder.	300 mg
Pantothenic acid	Part of Co-enzyme A, necessary for utilization of all energy-yielding nutrients.	Brewers' yeast. Dry milk or whey. Cane molasses. Alfalfa.	Synthetic calcium pantothenate (92% pantothenic acid).	2 g
Vitamin B_{12}	A cobalt-containing substance active in treating pernicious anaemia. Probably active part of "the animal protein factor".	Feeds of animal or marine origin. Liver meal is especially potent.	Fermentation products and byproducts from making antibiotics	5-10 mg for all young..

* Roughly equivalent to about one-fourth of the total needs of young animals (except for B_{12})

Minerals

With the increasing use of mineral supplements in the rations, it seems advisable to know the more common supplementary sources of these nutrients together with their composition.

Table : Sources of Minerals and Their Potency

Nutrient	Common source	Composition or potency	Remarks
Calcium	Feeding bone meal	26% Ca	Also contains 18% protein and 11% phosphorus.
	Feeding bone meal	29% Ca	Also contains 12% protein and 14% phosphorus.
	Bone char	27% Ca	Also contains 13% phosphorus but no protein
	Tricalcium phosphate	13% Ca	10% P
	Dicalcium phosphate	24% Ca	20% P
	Monocalcium phosphate	16% Ca	12% P
	Ground limestone	24-36% Ca	Balance likely to be carbonate and magnesium
	Calcium carbonate	40% Ca	
	Oyster and other marine shells	38% Ca	Shells contain on the average 96% $CaCO_3$
Phosphorus	Bone meals and Ca phosphates	(see above)	
	Rock phosphate	14% P	Rock phosphate is 75-80% tricalcium phosphate. Not advised unless guaranteed to contain less than 1% fluorine
	Defluorinated rock	18% P	Should not contain more than 1 part fluorine to 100 part phosphorus
Iodine	Potassium iodide	76% I	Potassium and sodium salts may be used interchangeably
	Sodium iodide	84% I	
	Potassium iodate	59% I	
	Iodize salt		Stabilized iodine should be used, Amounts of iodine differ but 0.02% and 0.05% are commonly sold

Iron	Ferric oxide	35% Fe	
	Ferrous sulphate	20% Fe	Originary copperas, commercial grade
	Reduced iron	80-100% Fe	May be 20% ferric oxide
Cobalt	Cobalt sulphate	34% Co	May be administered as a drench, as cobaltized salt, or as an ingredient in the ration

[a/] As source of calcium these products are useful in direct proportion to the calcium they contain

Non-Nutrient Feed Additives

Sweeteners, Binders and Flavours

Feed flavours are available in wide assortments. They are usually essential oils, whose distinctive aromas will permeate the feed into which they are mixed. Their presence can be detected months after the feeds are treated. It is often claimed that use of a flavouring material will aid digestion and stimulate appetite.

Antibiotics, Arsenicals and Nitro Furans

They have been found to possess the properties like bacteriostatic and bactericidal at effective levels having no toxic effect. In addition to their use as growth stimulants, these have been used at low levels to help protect feeds from microbial destruction and to prevent and control poultry diseases.

Anthelmetics

These are deworming drugs and used periodically in the feed or water to prevent parasitic infestation, specially of roundworms.

Antifungal

These are natural or synthetic substances which inhibit the growth of fungi.

Coccidiostat

These are routinely used in the diets of the poultry to prevent the most devastating type of disease the coccidiosis.

Pigmenters

These are usually the carotenoid sources added to feeds to improve pigmentation of broilers and egg-yolk.

Pellet Binders

These affect texture and firmness of pelleted feedstuffs.

Enzymes

These have shown under certain conditions to improve the digestibility of certain feed stuffs.

As regards to non-nutrient feed additives are concerned, no blanket recommendation is possible as to which additive is most useful. Here the nutritionist must decide which additive is most useful. Here the nutritionist must decide which feed additives are needed under each specific set of circumstances.

□□□

Chapter 18

Nutrient Requirement and Allowances

The requirement for a given nutrient is the minimum quantity of that nutrient, when all other nutrients are supplied in adequate quantities that will maintain normal growth and reproduction and, at the same time, prevent the development of symptoms of nutritional deficiency.

The accurate way to express the nutrient requirements is in amount per day per animal. Poultry are fed in groups. It is, therefore, not practical to express the requirements in amounts per day per animal. It is difficult to determine the needs of each member of the group according to the individual yield expected or to assess the effect on a bird of a reduction in the amount of a nutrient below the level at which the needs of all birds are satisfied. The nutrient requirements can be expressed in relation to energy content of the diet as poultry eat within limits to satisfy energy needs. The estimation of energy content of diet is not possible on routine basis and the calculated values may vary much from estimated values. Due to these difficulties the nutrient requirements of poultry are expressed on unit weight basis.

When the requirements are expressed on unit weight basis, voluntary feed intake (the amount of feed eaten by the bird) influences the nutrient requirements. Voluntary feed intake is dependent on size of the bird, energy content of diet, physical form of diet, nutritional adequacy of diet and environmental temperature.

The dietary allowance of a given nutrient is that quantity of the nutrient that is given to the animal. A reasonable allowance makes provision for a margin of safety. In most cases, allowances will exceed the requirements, for several reasons as listed below.

1. To provide a margin of safety
2. To allow for stability problem. Some nutrients are not stable for example several of fat-soluble vitamins are subjected to oxidative destruction
3. To allow for variations in composition of feed ingredients. These vary due to climatic conditions, variety of plant, fertilizer, etc.
4. To avoid loss during storage
5. To allow for increased concentration of the ration especially if added fat is used in the formulae
6. To allow for the nutrients destroyed in the digestive tract before they can accomplish their nutritional objectives.

Nutrient requirements of Turkey

S. No.	Nutrients	Turkey pre brooder feed (0-4 weeks)	Turkey brooder feed (5-8 weeks)	Turkey grower feed (9 -24 weeks)	Turkey breeder feed (above 24 weeks)
1	Energy (k.cal./kg feed	2800	2800	2700	2600
2	Crude protein (%)	28.00	26.00	21.00	14.00
3	Calcium (%)	1.30	1.10	1.00	2.30
4	Phosphorus (%)	1.00	0.50	0.40	0.40
5	Lysine (%)	1.70	1.60	1.20	1.00
6	Methionine (%)	0.50	0.50	0.40	0.40

NUTRIENTS	AGE (WEEKS)						
	TOM TURKEY						
	0-4	5-8	9-12	13-16	17-20	21-24	BREEDER TURKEY
	HEN TURKEY						
	0-4	5-8	9-11	12-14	15-17	18-20	
MINERALS							
Chlorine (%)	0.15	0.14	0.14	0.12	0.12	0.12	0.12
Magnesium (mg/kg)	600	600	600	600	600	600	600
Copper (mg/kg)	8	8	6	6	6	6	8
Iodine (mg/kg)	0.4	0.4	0.4	0.4	0.4	0.4	0.4
Iron (mg/kg)	80	60	60	60	50	50	60
Manganese (mg/kg)	60	60	60	60	60	60	60
Selenium (mg/kg)	0.2	0.2	0.2	0.2	0.2	0.2	0.2
Zinc (mg/kg)	75	65	50	40	40	40	65
VITAMINS							
FAT SOLUBLE VITAMINS							
Vitamin A (IU)	4000	4000	4000	4000	4000	4000	4000
Vitamin D3 (IU)	900	900	900	900	900	900	900
Vitamin E(IU)	12	12	10	10	10	10	25
Vitamin K(IU)	1	1	0.8	0.8	0.8	0.8	1
WATER SOLUBLE VITAMINS							
Biotine (mg/kg)	0.2	0.2	0.15	0.125	0.1	0.1	0.1
Choline (mg/kg)	1900	1600	1300	1100	950	800	1000
Folic acid (mg/kg)	1	1	0.8	0.8	0.7	0.7	1
Niacin (mg/kg)	70	70	50	50	40	40	40
Pantothenic acid (mg/kg)	11	11	9		9	9	16
Vitamin B2 (mg/kg)	3.6	3.6	3	3	2.5	2.5	4
Vitamin B1 (mg/kg)	2	2	2	2	2	2	2
Vitamin B6(mg/kg)	4.5	4.5	3.5	3.5	3	3	4
VITAMIN b12 (mg/kg)	0.003	0.003	0.003	0.003	0.003	0.003	0.003

The increase in the supply of the nutrient over the minimum over the minimum requirement is referred to as safety margin, the magnitude of which is dependent on the nature of nutrient. Minerals and vitamins constitute less than 10 per cent of the cost of diet and are more prone to destruction. For majority of the vitamins, usually twice the requirement is added as a safety margin, raising the total content of the nutrient in the diet to thrice the minimum requirement. The minimum requirements of trace minerals may be supplemented taking the amount present in the diet as safety margin. For major, 20 to 30 per cent of the minimum requirement is adequate as safety margin.

Several standards are available. The ones published now by the National Research Council (NRC) are the minimum requirements.

□□□

Chapter 19

Feed Formulation

The diets fed to poultry vary according to species, age and the purpose for which the stock are kept.

Most poultry feeds are

- Mash - Grind medium to fine,
- Pellets - Composed of mash feeds that are pelleted, and
- Crumbles - Produced by rolling pellets.

Pellets or crumbles - Cost slightly more, but can reduce feed wastage & sorting, readily adapted to automatic equipment, less feeder and storage space, and possibly improve palatability.

General Principles

- To find out the requirements of nutrients
- Whether the requirements will meet the productivity of the birds

- Quantity that will be consumed by the bird in a specific time
- Will this intake by the bird provide the requirements tabulated

Selecting Feedstuffs

- Nutrient availability - Affected by the fiber content, fat content, and amino acid balance.
- Palatability - Affected by the moisture content, contaminants
- Content of growth inhibitors or undesirable chemicals or pigments.
- Cost and market availability of feedstuffs.
- Digestibility

Information Required for Feed Formulation

- Requirements of nutrients for poultry and composition of a formulas in terms of nutrients
- Feed analytical values

The average nutrient content of the feed ingredient based on the analysis done previously available in the form of published table.

Maximum Level of Inclusion of Feed Ingredients

Inclusion of an ingredient beyond the maximum level may induce imbalance of nutrients, difficulty in feed formulation, may reduce the performance of the birds due to presence of antinutritional factors beyond tolerance level.

Availability and Cost of Feed Ingredients

- *Energy* - for poultry, metabolisable energy is considered. It is dependent on two basic assumptions i.e. that the metabolisable energy value of an ingredient is independent of other dietary components and that the value remains relatively constant regardless of age, type or nature of production of the bird.

Proteins and Amino Acids

The total protein requirement for poultry can be met easily. However it is difficult to meet the requirement for essential amino acids. Lysine and Methionine are the limiting amino acids in our practical acids. There fore, the amino acid requirement can be restricted in practical feed formulation to the requirement of lysine and methionine.

Minerals and Vitamins

Steps in Feed Formulation

In practical diet formulation by calculation, the essential steps are as follows: The ingredients are added to the formula to provide the nutrients per kg or 100 kg or 1000 kg diet.

- Start by satisfying the protein requirements, both for quantity and quality (amounts of essential amino acids).
- The levels of animal protein sources are fixed. These are added at fixed levels because of cost.
- The level of cereal by-products if to be added may be fixed.
- Vegetable protein sources and energy sources are added to provide the required amount of protein.
- The metabolisable energy content of the diet has to be balanced. The shortfall if any can be met by supplementation of fats and oils.
- Balance the protein and energy contents. Keep the ratio of calories to protein in line with the needs of the birds. Try to stay within two percent of the ratio. The number or ratio is useful only as a guideline in checking if there is enough protein in the feed.
- Calculate the total crude fiber content of the feed. Try to keep it below five percent.
- The phosphorus content of the diet is calculated in terms of available phosphorus. Phosphorus from animal and inorganic sources is considered completely available, whereas that from plant sources is considered to be 30 per cent available.
- The calcium content of the diet is calculated. The shortfall in calcium requirement can be met by the addition of limestone. Keep the calcium/phosphorus ratio in the recommended range.
- The limiting amino acids (lysine and methionine) in synthetic form can be supplemented to meet the protein requirement.

- Balancing the vitamin and-mineral contents of feed. To meet the needs add a commercial vitamin-mineral supplement. If the supplement's directions are followed the, the birds get enough of their needs without any harmful excesses.
- A check is made for the total of the ingredients and also for all the nutrients if desired.

Mixing the feed ingredients

Different ingredients are mixed as per the formula to make the complete diet. Ingredients like maize and groundnut-cake are ground before mixing. For chicks during early part, fine grinding is necessary. Later, medium grinding may be adequate. After addition of all ingredients usually 10- 15 minutes of time is allowed depending on the mixer. Ingredients added in small quantity such as trace minerals, vitamins and other feed additives are premixed prior to addition in the mixer. The size of the premix may be 250 g to 1.5 kg per 100 kg diet.

Suggested feed formulation for turkeys suitable for indian climatic conditions

Ingredients (kg)	Turkey pre brooder mash (0-4 weeks)	Turkey brooder mash (5 to 8 weeks)	Turkey grower feed (9-24 weeks)	Turkey layer feed (above 24 weeks)
Maize	44	47	43	41
Deoiled rice bran	-	-	22	24
Soya bean meal	45	36	14.5	13.5
Sunflower oil cake	-	7	11.5	9
Dry fish	9.5	9	8	8
Mineral mixture	0.5	0.5	0.5	1.5
Dicalcium phosphate	1	0.5	0.5	-
Calcite powder	-	-	-	-
Shell grit	-	-	-	3
Total	100	100	100	100

Inclusion level and nutrient content of commonly used feed ingredients

Feed ingredient	Inclusion level %	Crude protein %	Energy (kcal/kg)	Lysine %	Methionine %	Calcium %	Phosphorus %
Maize	0-60	9.00	3370	0.20	0.20	0.03	0.10
Sorghum	0-40	10.00	3260	0.20	0.20	0.04	0.10
Cumbu	0-40	12.00	2880	0.40	0.20	0.07	0.20
Broken rice	0-30	9.00	3090	0.10	0.10	0.04	0.02
Wheat	0-50	10.00	3100	0.30	0.20	0.10	0.10
Rice bran	0-20	14.00	2890	0.60	0.20	0.07	1.60
sunflower oil cake	0-15	27.00	1900	1.10	0.70	0.10	0.10
groundnut oil cake	0-20	45.00	2420	1.50	0.42	0.23	0.54
Soya bean meal	0-40	44.00	2420	3.00	0.60	0.30	0.30
Fish meal	10-15	45.00	2460	3.90	1.20	8.00	2.00
Molasses	5-10	3.00	2000	-	-	0.10	0.10
Mineral mixture	2-3	-	-	-	-	30.00	6.00
Vegetable oil	0-5	-	-	-	-	-	-

□□□

Chapter 20

Feeding Turkeys

The turkey continues to show improved market performance in terms of weight for age and feed efficiency.

Feeding Marketing Turkeys

Change diets frequently to adjust to the specific needs and to minimize feed costs. They grow faster than chickens, thus have relatively higher requirements. Protein requirements decrease by age - 28% with starting poults to 16 % for mature birds. Energy requirements tend to increase during the growing stage ranging from 2,900 to 3,300 kcal/kg. Upon arrival, poults should be encouraged to consume feed and water as soon as possible - Using coloured plastic feed plates or placing brightly colored marbles in the feed and water. Antibiotic & coccidiostat - may be necessary for early starter diets but once past 8 to 12 weeks of age, optional. Marketing- Males/toms - 18 to 20 wk of age & 4- 4.5 kg live weight. Females/hens - 16 to 18 week of age and about 3-3.5 kg live weight.

Feeding Holding and Breeding Turkeys

Feed the holding diet from 16 to 18 week of age until the beginning of the lighting program (2 week before egg production), which usually occurs about 30 week of age. Holding diet - Contains less energy than the starter and grower diets & delays sexual maturity, which may result in desirable effects on later reproductive performance. After 30 week or so of age, feed the breeder diet. Breeder females can be provided a diet with 14% protein and 2600 kcal/kg energy. Toms can be provided with 12-13% protein.

Performance of Beltsville small white turkey under Indian conditions (Average feed intake/bird, average body weight/bird and feed conversion ratio)

Age in weeks	Average feed intake (g)	Average body weight(g)	FCR
Upto 4	650	270	2.40
Upto 8	2670	970	2.75
Upto 12	5010	1545	3.25
Upto 16	7880	2245	3.50
Upto 20	11080	2885	3.80
Upto 24	14700	3475	4.25

❑❑❑

Chapter 21

Nutritional Deficiencies

The definite diagnosis of nutritional deficiencies in poultry requires experienced technicians and sophisticated pathology laboratory facilities. This is because:

- Deficiency symptoms are not noticed until severe.
- Symptoms of any specific nutrient deficiency are similar to symptoms of non-nutritional diseases and/or other deficiencies.

Vitamins

Vitamins	Deficiency symptoms
A	Retarded growth, nutritional group, bleached beak and shanks, staggering gait.
Thiamin (B_1)	Retarded growth, emaciation, retraction of head
Pyridoxine	Retarded growth, convulsions

D	Retarded growth, rickets, soft-shelled eggs. Decreased egg production and hatchability
E	"Crazy-chick" disease (Nutritional Ence phalomalacia) Loss of fertility in males, decreased hatchability
Biotin	Incrustations in bottom of feet.
K	Haemorrhages
Riboflavin (B_2)	Retarded growth, decreased, hatchability, "Curledtoe" paralysis
Pantothenic acid	Incrustations at corners of mouth and on the upper surface of the feet
Folic acid	Poor growth, feather development and hatchability
Choline	Perosis or slipped tendon
B_{12}	Very poor growth and decreased hatchability
Niacin	Black tongue condition

Minerals

Minerals	Deficiency symptoms
Calcium	Retarded growth, soft bones, decreased egg production and hatchability; thin shells.
Phosphorous	Retarded growth, soft bones, decreased egg production
Manganese	Slipped tendon or perosis, thin-shelled or shell-less eggs; decreased hatchability; abnormal embryoa
Zinc	Retarded growth;enlarge-ment of hock joint; scaling of skin; poor feathering shortening and thickening of leg bones
Iron, Copper	Anaemia,aorta rupture; feather depigmentation
Iodine	Enlargement of thyroid; loweredrate of body activity; impaired physical, mental response
Magnesium	Slow growth,lethargic;loss of appetite; stalled chicks show evidence of spasm and shock, and become prostrate
Selenium	Exudative diathesis, muscular dystrophy
Sodium, Potassium	Retarded growth of soft tissues and muscles.

□□□

Chapter 22

Guidelines for the Establishment of a Feed Mill

The design and location of a feed mill should be guided by the customers it is to serve with important consideration given to soil conditions and whether or not an area is prone to flooding. It is important that the mill be located so that any impacts from wet conditions are minimized and the area kept free of heavy undergrowth and bushes. It is equally important that local transportation infrastructure be utilized to the extent that railway spurs, wharves, and highways are considered for receipt of raw ingredients and also for the ease and cost-effectiveness with which the farmers are to receive their feed.

Areas prone to flooding, tidal inundation, and fire should be avoided if at all possible. It is important to remember that if the mill cannot deliver feed on schedule due to flood or other natural disaster the feed miller is not the only one at risk, but it may put the farmer at risk as well. It is important to locate the plant such that future expansion of mill facilities can be accomplished cost-effectively. Initially, the mill equipment should be sized and designed to allow for expansion and easy change of equipment as new techniques in milling evolve and/or the culture species change. Flexibility in the mill design is vital if one is to remain competitive.

Safety and hygiene factors should be built into the plant design. Buildings should be designed to prevent the entrance and harboring of vermin and birds. Cleaning and maintenance of all buildings and the avoidance of uncleanable recesses should be considered in the design and construction and in the selection of materials. The property should be configured to contain and/or manage any spills or runoff from the mill site. In wet areas elevator and receiving pits should have drains (and/or sump pumps) to prevent flooding. It is important, too, that the plant be a good commercial neighbor, that by design it is inoffensive and a positive force in the community, complying with local health, safety, and environmental regulations and always presents a clean and neat appearance. Regular inspections by management are important to assure the good outward appearance and a high standard of cleanliness, as well as to be certain that all equipment is performing to specification.

Strategy

A.	The Concept	B.	Requirements of a feed Mill	C.	Planning the Project
A.1	Type of Factory	B.1	Production	C.1	Phase One - Inception
A.2	Marketing Appreciation	B.1.1	Material handling	C.1.1	The feasibility study team
A. 2.1	Product list	B.1.1.1	Weighbridge for both deliveries and dispatches	C.1.1.1	The project team
A.2.2	Target turnovers	B.1.1.2	Adequate handling facilities for rapid material flow	C.1.1.2	The manageme nt team
A.3	Costs and Capital Requirements	B.1.1.3	Adequate storage space for bulk and sacked materials	C.1.2	Primary considerations
A.3.1	Amount capital required	B.1.2	Product manufacturing	C.1.2.1	Market analysis
A.3.2	Sources of capital	B.1.2.1	Size reduction	C.1.2.2	Availability of raw materials

A.4	Development and Other Grants	B.1.2.2	Conveying	C.1.2.3	Labour
A.5	Location	B.1.2.3	Mixing	C.1.2.4	Transport and communications
A.5.1	Proximity to markets	B.1.2.4	Pelleting and crumblizing	C.1.2.5	Political issues
A.5.2	Proximity to raw materials	B.1.2.5	Bagging-off	C.1.2.6	Technical and process know-how
A.5.3	Other considerations	B.1.3	Warehouse	C.1.2.7	Contractual procedures
A.6	Availability of Labour	B.1.3.1	Protection from elements	C.1.3	Outcome of phase one
A.7	Raw Materials	B.1.3.2	Rodent and insect pests control	C.1.3.1	Decision on parameters considered
A.7.1	Local	B.1.4	Laboratory	C.1.3.2	Definition of responsibilities of various personalities involved in both teams
A.7.2	Imports	B.1.4.1	Raw material check	C.2	Phase Two - 'The Brief'
A.8	Transport and Communications	B.1.4.2	Product quality control	C.2.1	Precise instructions to project team from management team
A.9	Public Services	B.1.4.3	New product development	C.2.1.1	Preparation of lay-out drawings
A.9.1	Electrical power	B.2	Technical and Engineering	C.2.1.2	Detailed report on all elements of the project
A.9.2	Fuel oil	B.2.1	Building	C.3	Phase Three - Design

Equipment Requirements for 8-Ton-an-hour Feed Mill

Item	Quantity	HP each motor	Size and Capacity
Receiving			
Truck Hoist	1	10	8 ton
Power Shovel	1	3	-
Conveyor, drag	1	5	9 in × 45 ft
Elevator, bucket	1	10	8 in × 5 in bucket
Magnet, plate	1	-	8 in
Scalper	1	1	25 t/h
Distributor	1	¼	10 positions
Storage tanks	2	-	5 000 gal
Diverter valve	1		8 in

Hammermill	1	60	8-12 t/h
Elevator, bucket	1	2	8 in × 5 in bucket
Diverter valve	1	-	8 in
Mixing			
Feeder conveyor	9	3-2, 6 -3	
Feeder, loading board	1	-	-
Weigh hopper and scale	1	-	120 cu ft
Vertical mixer with surge bin	2	7 ½	100 cu ft each
Conveyor, screw	1	3	12 in × 20 ft
Elevator, bucket	1	7 ½	8 in × 5 in bucket
Continuous mixer	1	5	5 t/h
Molasses pump, heating		7	
tank and other		5 ½	
equipment	1		10 gal/min
Fat system	1	3	10 gal/min
Diverter valve	1	-	8 in
Pelleting			
Pellet mill	1	75,5, ½	7-10 t/hr
Cooler, fan collector	1	20 ½	7-10 t/hr
Crumbler	1	10	6 in × 60 in
Scalper	1	1	60 in × 72 in
Elevators, buckets	2	1	8 in × 15 ft
Distributor	1	3 ¼	8 in × 30 ft 8 hole
Packing			
Scale belt feeder	1	¾	7 × 50 lb/min
Bag conveyor	1	1	7 bags/min
Sewing machine	1	1/3	7 bags/min
Warehousing			
Forklift	1	-	3 000 lb
Bulk Loadant			
Conveyor, drag	1	5	12 in × 30 ft
Travel weigh hopper	1	1	3 t
Miscellaneous			
Boiler	1	1	150 hp
Air compressor	1	1	-
Control panel	1	1	-

[1/] Adapted from "Feed Manufacturing Costs and Capital Requirements" ERS-USDA, Agricultural Economic Report No. 335, 1976

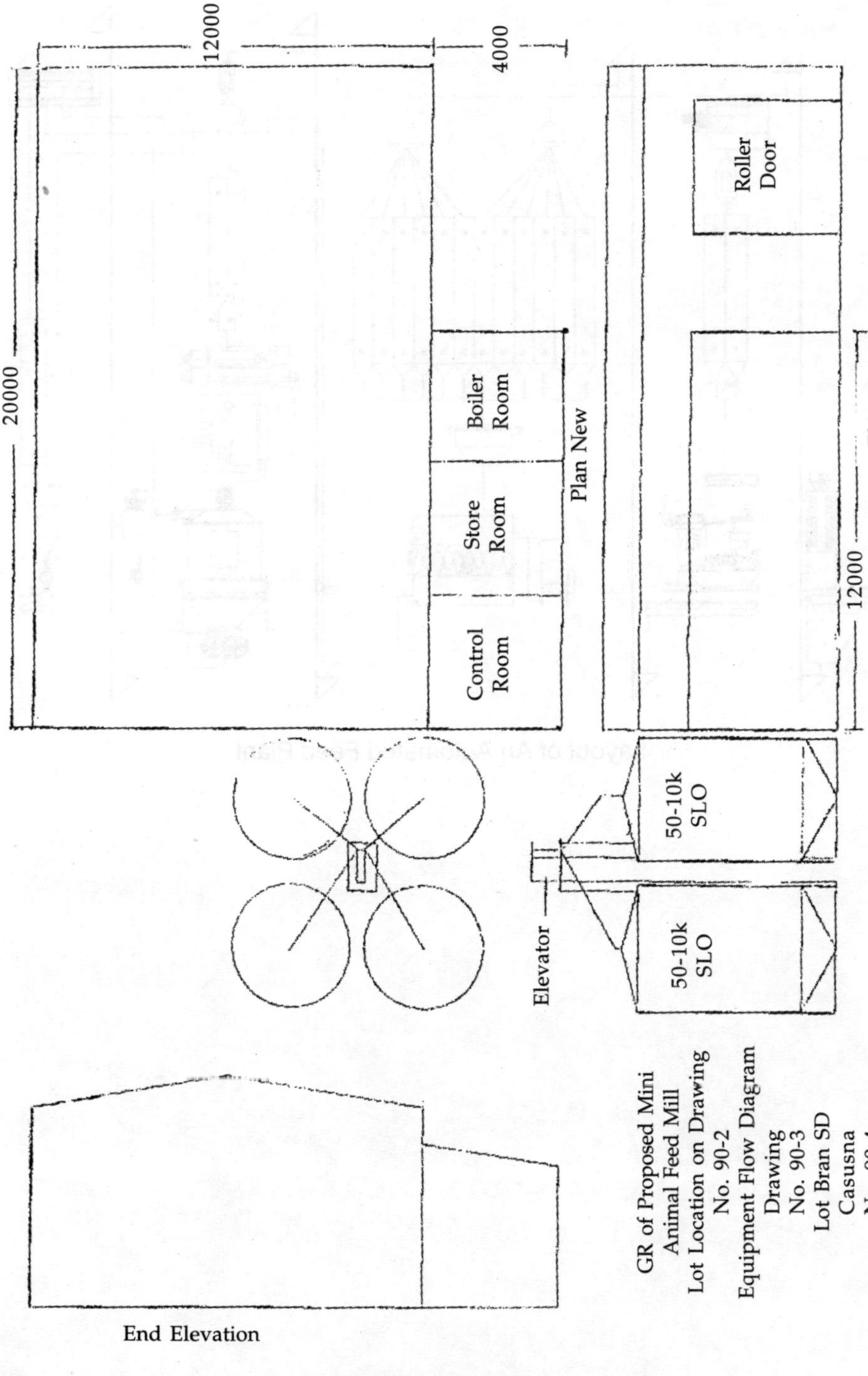

Layout of a Feed Mill

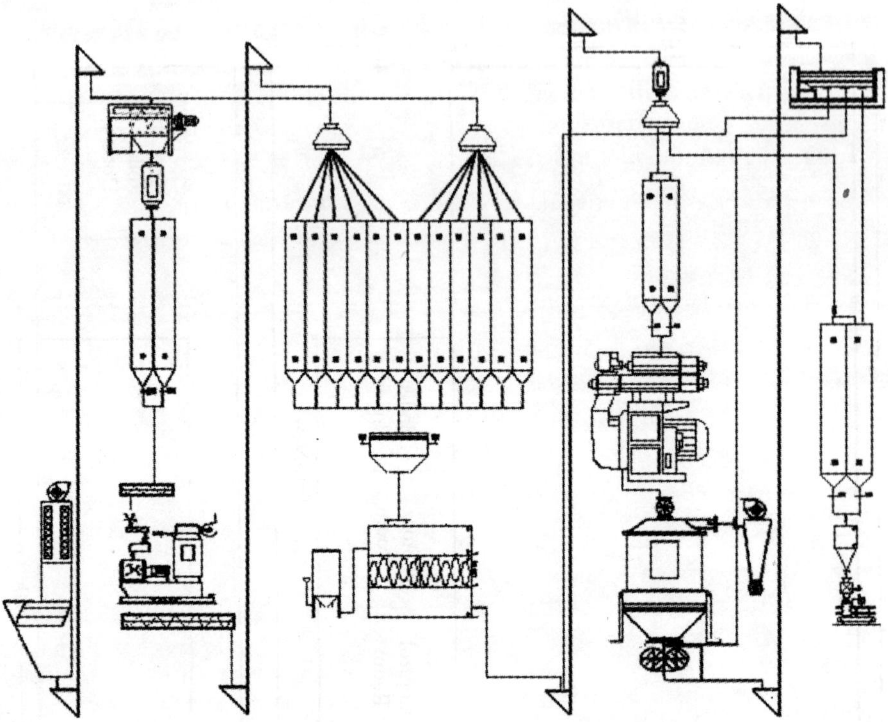

Layout of An Automated Feed Plant

Chapter 23

Material Flow in Feed Manufacturing

Introduction

The technology of feed processing has undergone substantial improvement in recent years. It was only sixty years ago that feeds tuffs were mixed on the warehouse floor by the use of a shovel. Feed processing has progressed from the simple mixing of several ingredients by hand to mechanical mixing, to continuous mixing, and now to computer controlled mixing and pelleting. However, the basic concept of mixing ingredients together to result in a nutritionally balanced feed, has remained unchanged.

To accomplish the mixing of different ingredients, grinding these ingredients to similar particle sizes, and then putting them together in a single unit, requires a considerable amount of specialized equipment and technical expertise. Some feed plants are designed for specific functions, such as making poultry feeds exclusively; others are designed for producing a variety of feeds. Regardless of the specific purpose of a feed plant, material flow follows a basic pattern.

Receiving

The first operation in the feed processing plant involves the receiving of raw materials into the plant premises. Feed ingredients arrive in sacks, or other small containers, and in bulk.

Sacked ingredients are checked for identification and condition. They are then logged in after segregation of drugs and medications. Sacked ingredients must then be stored in a dry location with proper protection from rodent and insect infestation. Sacked stocks are then rotated to minimize staleness, product degradation, and insect infestation.

Bulk ingredients are handled according to their physical form. Liquid ingredients, such as oils and molasses, are generally stored in bulk tanks. Proper storage temperature is maintained and the filter screens are checked periodically. Solid bulk ingredients such as grains, oil meals, etc., are cleaned with a scalper to remove foreign material prior to storage in bins. Bin temperatures are monitored to prevent heating due to grinning respiration.

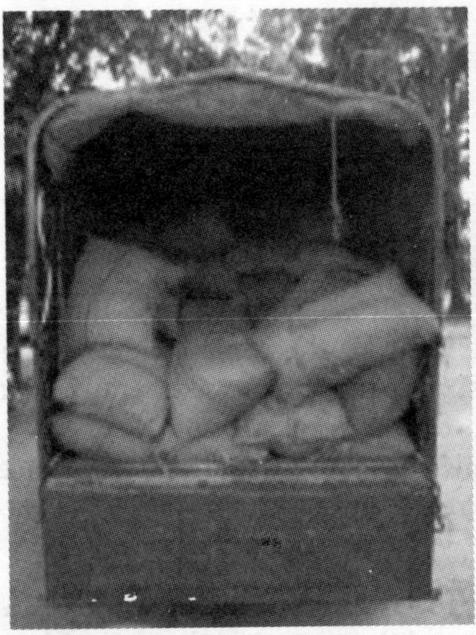

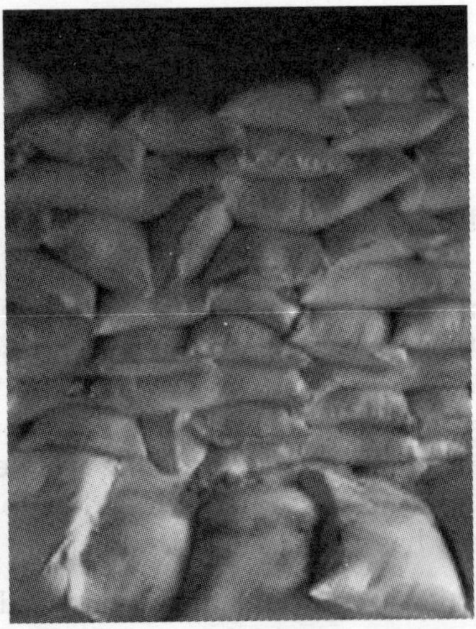

Processing

Material flow during processing includes:

(a) Particle size reduction
(b) Premixing

(c) Mixing
(d) Pelleting and
(e) Sacking

Coarse ingredients pass over a permanent magnet which removes tramp metal and then through a hammer mill which reduces particle size to the desired screen analysis. Ground material is monitored periodically to ensure size uniformity and to help detect wear of hammer mill screen and hammers. The ground material is then routed to ingredient holding bins.

There are two mixing operations in feed milling. One is for the mixing of micro-nutrients; the operation is generally termed pre-mixing. The other mixing operation involves the actual blending of all components of the diet.

Micro-nutrients, such as vitamins and trace minerals, are accurately weighed with carrier material which has a density approximating that of the predominant micro-ingredient. The materials are then mixed in a batch mixer for a period of time specified by the equipment manufacturer to ensure homogeneity. The premix is finally routed to the premix holding bin.

Diet mixing begins when augers are set in motion to deliver; the correct amounts of each ingredient including the premix, according to the formula, into the mixer. Where manual changing of the mixer is done, ingredients are weighed out in sacks or hopper carts. The mixing period is according to the equipment manufacturer's specifications, but final mix is checked periodically with a tracer to ensure homogeneity of the mix. If the mixed diet is to undergo pelleting, it is routed to the pelleting bin.

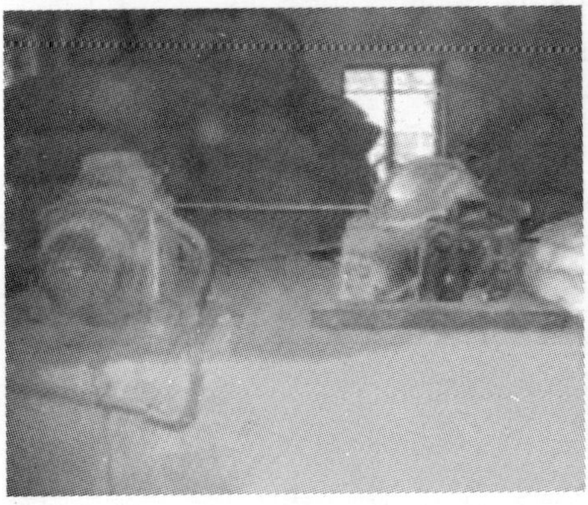

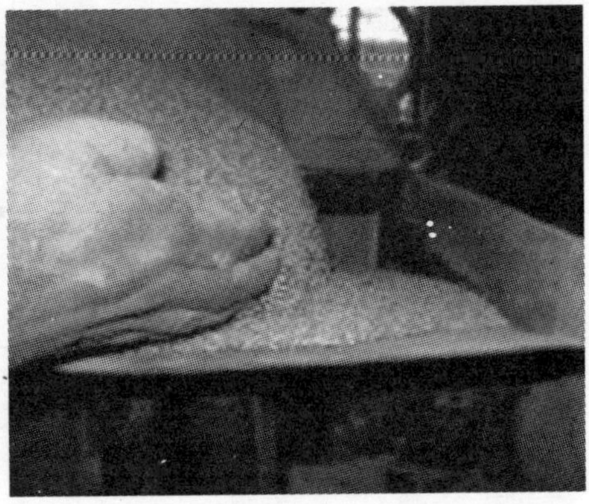

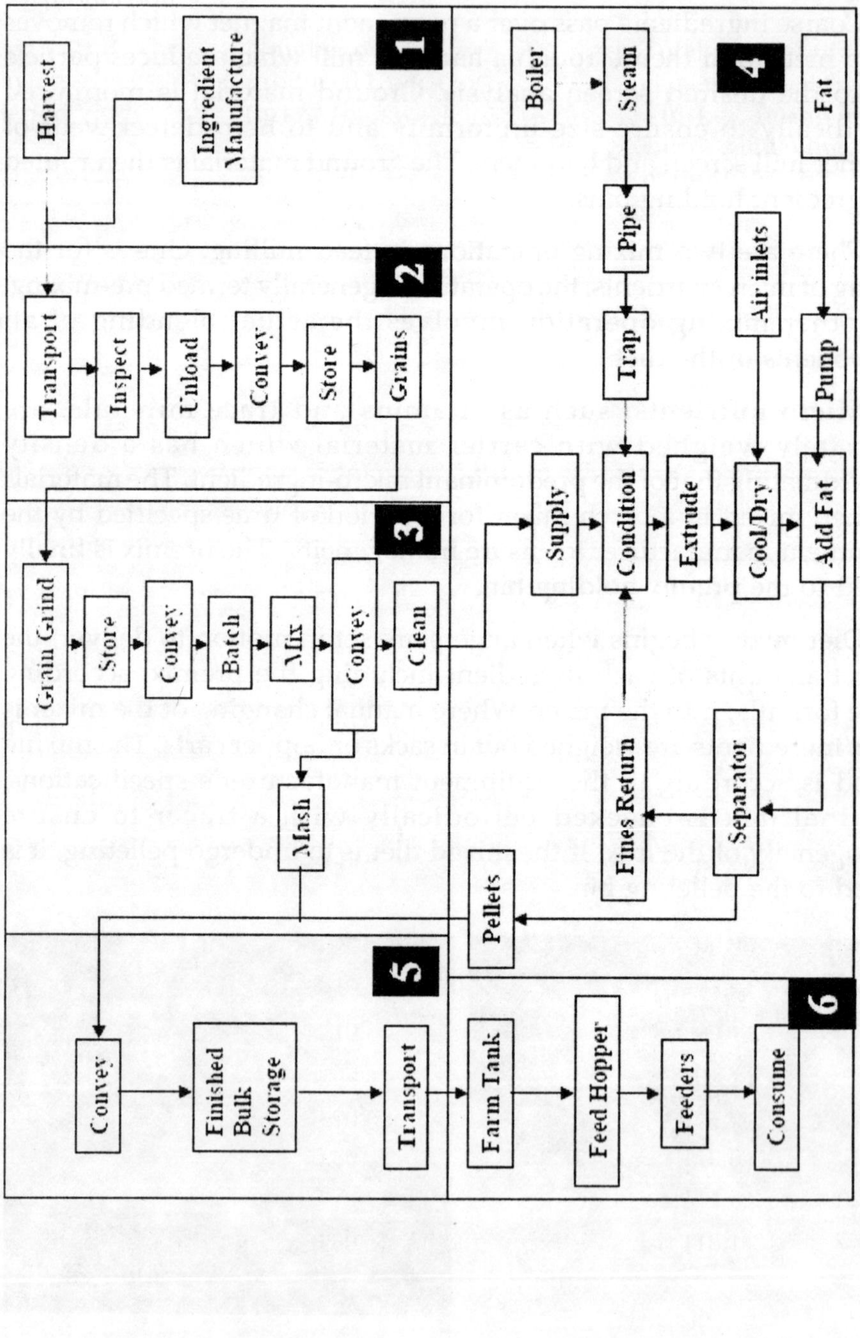
1
Harvest
Ingredient Manufacture
2
Transport
Inspect
Unload
Convey
Store
Grains
3
Grain Grind
Store
Convey
Batch
Mix
Convey
Clean
Mash
4
Boiler
Steam
Pipe
Trap
Supply
Condition
Extrude
Cool/Dry
Air inlets
Fat
Pump
Add Fat
Fines Return
Separator
Pellets
5
Convey
Finished Bulk Storage
Transport
6
Farm Tank
Feed Hopper
Feeders
Consume

Flow Chart

Mixed feed mash for pelleting is first conditioned with steam in the steam conditioner section of the pellet mill, after which it enters the die where it is finally extruded. Freshly extruded pellets are hot and contain excess moisture which is removed during passage through the cooler. Fines are then screened from the cooled pelleted feed and returned for repeating. Fish oil, if added, is now applied prior to the routing of the finished pellets into the packer bins.

Packaging

Most fish feed pellets are sacked. The sacking operation includes: weighing, sacking, taping, coding, and sewing. The sacked bags are then sent to the warehouse for distribution.

Storage and Distribution

Bulk products are stored in large bins. Feed is loaded into specially constructed bulk carriers and delivered to the customer. Feed is discharged from the truck into customer storage facility by means of an auger system, paddle conveyor, or pneumatic system.

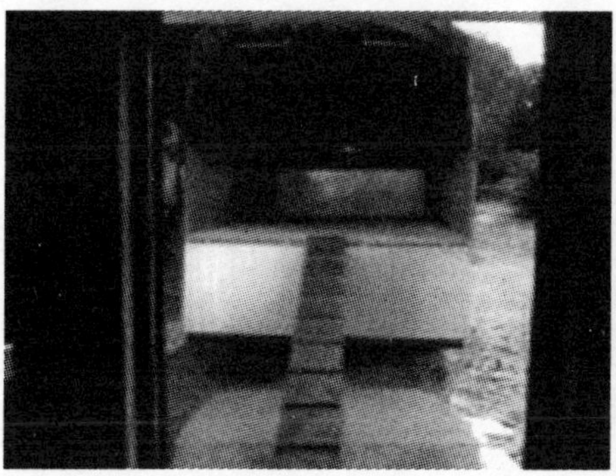

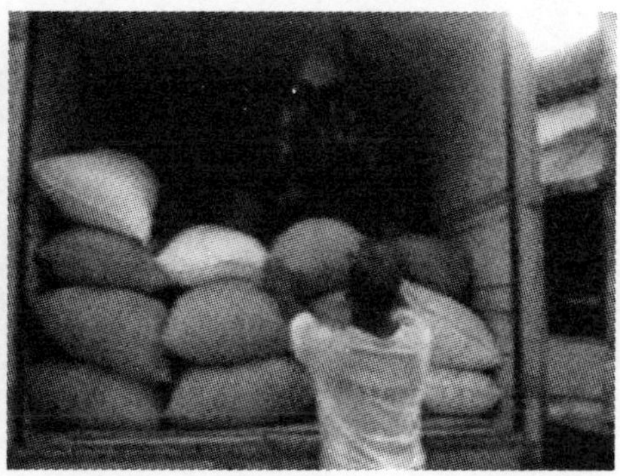

□□□

Chapter 24

Feed Milling Processes

Introduction

Feed manufacturing and the associated quality control programme are keys to successful poultry farming. Unless the poultry nutritionist understands and specifies the activities of the feed mill and its laboratory, profitable poultry farming will be a matter of chance.

Dry feeds may be ground, sifted, screened, mixed, compressed, expanded, texturized, coloured and flavoured. By one or more of these processes, a wide variety of ingredients can be prepared into a standardized product. Since most fish have size and texture preferences and often react to colour, odour, and flavour, processing research is an integral part of poultry farming.

Grinding

Grinding or particle-size reduction is a major function of feed manufacturing. Many feed mills pass all incoming ingredients through a grinder for several reasons:

(a) Clumps and large fragments are reduced in size,

(b) Some moisture is removed due to aeration, and

(c) Additives such as antioxidants may be blended.

All of these improve the ease of handling ingredients and their storability.

There are other reasons for grinding and the associated sieving of ingredients in formula feeds before further processing. Extremes in particle sizes are wasteful and often dangerous. The grinding of ingredients generally improves feed digestibility, acceptability, mixing properties, pelletability, and increases the bulk density of some ingredients. It is accomplished by many types of manual and mechanical operations involving impact, attrition, and cutting.

Hammer Mills

Hammer mills are mostly impact grinders with swinging or stationary steel bars forcing ingredients against a circular screen or solid serrated section designated as a striking plate. Material is held in the grinding chamber until it is reduced to the size of the openings in the screen. The number of hammers on a rotating shaft, their size, arrangement, sharpness, the speed of rotation, wear patterns, and clearance at the tip relative to the screen or striking plate are important variables in grinding capacity and the appearance of the product. Heat imparted to the material, due to the work of grinding, is related to the time it is held within the chamber and the air flow characteristics. Impact grinding is most efficient with dry, low-fat ingredients, although many other materials may be reduced in size by proper screen selection and regulated intake.

Most hammer mills have a horizontal drive shaft which suspends vertical hammers but for some ingredients, such as dried animal byproducts, a "vertical" hammer mill is more efficient. In this mill, the drive shaft is positioned vertically and screens and hammers are positioned horizontally. Material successfully reduced in size to the diameter of screen holes or smaller, is carried by gravity outside the mill and thence by air or conveyor to storage in "make-up" bins. Oversize particles, not easily broken, drop through the mill and may be recycled or discarded. Thus foreign materials, such as metal and stones, are discharged before they are forced through the screen causing damage.

Hammer Mill

The reduction of grain into small particles using a hammer mill is determined by the number of hammers, hammer size, hammer wear, hammer tip speed, tractor horsepower, screen area, the diameter of the screen opening, grinding rate (rate at which grain is fed to the grinder), and grain quality (moisture, hardness, grain test weight/ bulk density, grain type).The hammer number and dimensions are usually determined by the manufacturer of the portable grinder-mixer.

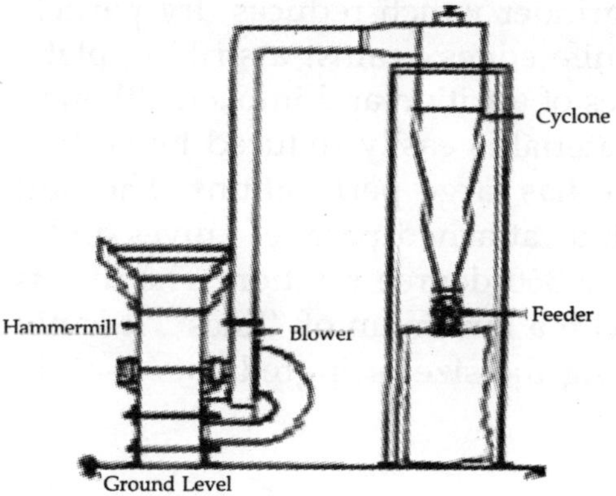

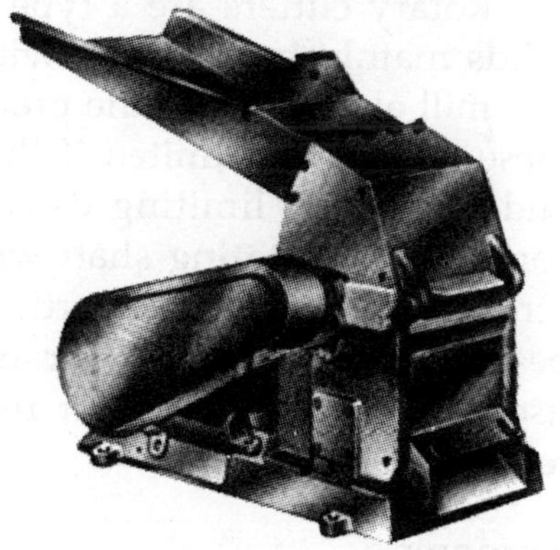

Attrition Mills

Attrition mills use the hammer mill principle to a certain extent; i.e., shattering by/impact. However, they also impart a shearing and cutting action. Grinding is done between two discs equipped with replaceable wearing surfaces. One or both of these discs is rotated; if both, they rotate in opposite directions. When one disc is rotated, and the other stationary, the assembly is used for shredding and deferring. Often materials which have been coarsely ground by other mills are passed through an attrition mill for blending or smoothing out an ingredient or mixture containing liquids which may have clumps. The discs of an attrition mill are generally in a vertical position so that materials not capable of reduction can pass by gravity out of the grinding area.

Roller Mills

A combination of cutting, attrition, and crushing occurs in roller mills. These are smooth or corrugated rolls rotating at the same speed set at a pre-determined distance apart with material passing between the two. A tearing action may be added by operating the rolls at different speeds and by corrugations which are different for each roll; i.e., the top roll may have off-radial spiral corrugations and the bottom roll lateral corrugations. This last type, called a "Le Page cut" is used in making granules from hard pellets, as it provides a breaking surface without much impact to cause dust. Roll grinding is economical but limited to materials which are fairly dry and low in fat.

Cutters

Rotary cutters are a type of grinder which reduces dry particle solids mainly by shearing with knife edges against a striking plate. The mill also includes the processes of attrition and impact, although these actions are limited if the material is easily reduced by cutting and the screen limiting discharge has large perforations. The mill consists of a rotating shaft with four attached parallel knives and a screen occupying one fourth of the 360 degree rotation. The mill is best used to crack whole grains with a minimum of "fines". It is not used as a final process for reducing the size of ingredients used in feeds.

Screening

Associated with grinding feeds, a sieving system is required which classifies materials to any desired particle size. The "overs" in this system may be re-ground or rejected. The "throughs" may be selected to comply with fish preferences for size and mixed according to formula specifications. Hammer mill or impact grinding of dry feeds, especially cereal grains, creates particles within the range called "dust", and a dust-collecting system may be necessary to remove this. An excess of dust in the feed may lead to gill disease, a situation where organic matter adhering to gills becomes a nutrient for bacteria or parasites.

The problem of excess dust formed by grinding feeds may be partly alleviated by adding a spray of oil or a semi-moist ingredient, such as condensed fish solubles or fermentation solubles, on feeds entering the grinder. Dehydrated alfalfa is prepared as a dust-free meal, similar in texture to a sifted crumblized pellet, by spraying mineral oil into a hammer mill chamber during grinding.

Mixing

The objective of feed mixing is to start with a certain assortment of ingredients called a "formula", totalling some definite weight. This is processed so that each small unit of the whole, either a mouthful or a day's feeding, is the same proportion as the original formula. Mixing is recognized as an empirical unit operation, which means that it is more of an art than a science and must be learned by experience.

Feed mixing may include all possible combinations of solids and liquids. Within each ingredient are differences in physical properties. For solids there are differences in particle size, shape, density, electrostatic charge, coefficient of friction as represented by the angle of repose, elasticity or resilience and, of course, colour, odour, and taste. For liquids there are differences in viscosity and density.

Mixing may be either a batch or a continuous process. Batch mixing can be done on an open flat surface with shovels or in containers shaped as cylinders, half-cylinders, cones or twin-cones with fixed baffles or moving augers, spirals, or paddles. Continuous mixing proportions by weight or volume, is a technique best suited for formula feeds with few ingredients and minimal changes.

Horizontal Mixers

Continuous Ribbon Mixers

The continuous or "twin-spiral" mixer consists of a horizontal, stationary, half-cylinder with revolving helical ribbons placed on a central shaft so as to move materials from one end to the other as the shaft and ribbon rotate inside. Capacity can be from a few litres to several cubic metres. The speed of shaft rotation will vary inversely as the circumference of the outer ribbon; usually optimum between 75-100 metres per minute. Since material travel is from one end to the other, either end may be used for discharge. These mixers may be inverted for cleaning.

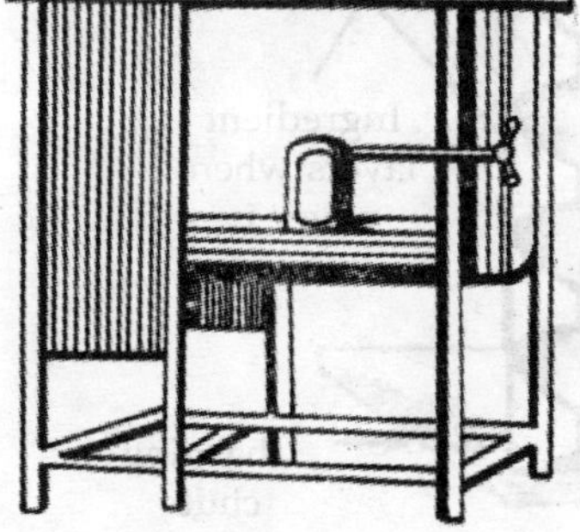

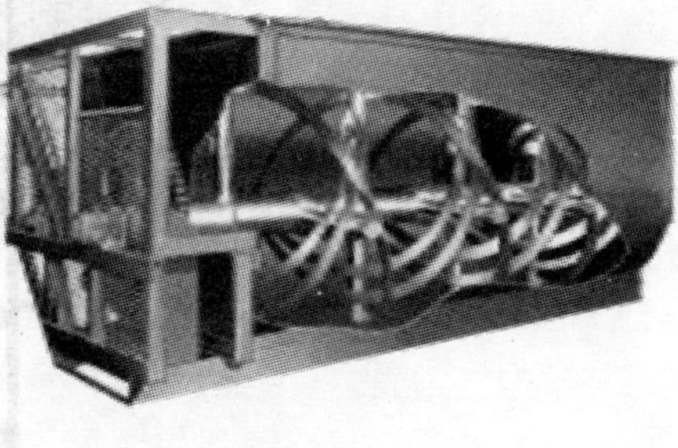

Non-Continuous Ribbon Mixers

Non-continuous or interrupted ribbons are similar to the continuous ribbon mixers except that short sections called "paddles" or "ploughs" are spaced in a spiral round the mixer shaft. Action is different from that of continuous ribbon mixers, and may be more satisfactory for mixing liquids with dry solids. These mixers are made in a wide variety of sizes with travel of the outer diameter of paddles from 100 to 120 metres per minute.

Continuous Ribbon Mixer

Vertical Mixers

Vertical mixers may consist of a cylinder, cone, or hopper-shaped container, with a single or double screw (auger) located vertically through the centre. The screw operates at speeds of 100 to 200 rpm and vertically conveys incoming materials from the bottom (generally the intake) end, like a screw conveyor, to the top where they are scattered and fall by gravity. This sequence is repeated several times until a blend is attained (usually from 10 to 12 minutes). These mixers may also be loaded from the top. Results show that vertical mixers are not efficient for uniform mixing of solids and liquids or for materials of quite different particle size or density. This unit is difficult to clean and there may be inter-batch contamination.

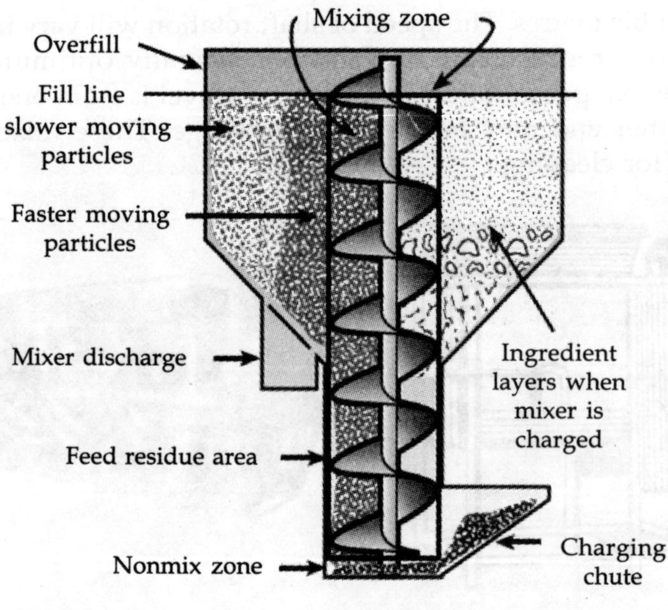

Pelleting

The transformation of a soft, often dusty feed into a hard pellet is accomplished by compression, extrusion, and adhesion. The general process involves passing a feed mixture through a conditioning chamber where 4 to 6 percent water (usually as steam) may be added. Moisture provides lubrication for compression and extrusion and in the presence of heat causes some gelatinization of raw starch present on the surface of vegetative ingredients, resulting in adhesion. Within 20 seconds of entering the pellet mill, feed goes from an air-dry (about 10-12 percent moisture) condition at ambient temperature, to 15-16 percent moisture at 80-90°C. During subsequent compression and extrusion through holes in a ring' die, friction further increases feed temperature to nearly 92°C. Pellets discharged onto a screen belt of a horizontal tunnel drier or into a vertical screened hopper are air-cooled within 10 minutes to slightly above ambient temperatures and dried to below 13 percent moisture.

Contrary to early belief, finished pellets contain practically all the nutrients found in feedstuffs and additives as compounded. The loss of thermo labile vitamins used in additives, which may be slight or extensive in the case of vitamin C, may be compensated for by extra supplementation of these in the vitamin premix to comply with formula requirements. Diastatic enzymes (alpha and beta amylase) present in whole grains and cereal byproducts are still active after processing by grinding and pelleting, although powdered enzymes added as an ingredient are inactivated.

Packaging and Labelling

Packaging

Poultry feeds are usually packed in gunny bags/woven polypropylene (PP) bags 50 kg with no inner lining. All feed bags are sealed by stitching manually or mechanically.

- The function of packaging is to protect the finished feed from light and moisture and other environmental contaminants. Together with labelling, it should tell the farmer the identity of the manufacturer and the type of feed it is.
- The feed label describes the contents of the sack or package and the species for which it is intended. For bulk feed, that which may be delivered in quantity as by truck, or sea container, the label and instructions for application of the feed should be attached to the invoice.

- If the feed is medicated, warnings should be clearly evident along with specific instructions for the species being fed.

Details of what must be accomplished for packaging and labelling of finished feed should include:

Bagging

- The sack-off operator should check and clean all equipment before bagging;
- Scales should be tested for accuracy, including bag tare;
- Verify bags and/or tags are properly coded for the day's run;
- At the beginning of a bagging run, initial bags of a new feed may need to be set aside until proper consistency of product quality is observed. The feed in these bag(s) may be medicated the mill superintendent should be consulted before re-running the feed; all bags should be properly labelled, including instructions for feeding the species to be fed; and
- At the beginning and throughout every run, bags should be periodically check-weighed; and all scales must be certified annually.

Labels and Tags

Labels and feed tags will conform to the law published by the jurisdiction in which the turkey feed products are being sold.

It should be the responsibility of the feed mill manager to

- Co-ordinate the layout and printing of tags;
- Check the tags for accuracy and government compliance before tags are printed in quantity;
- Labels should be received, handled and stored in a manner that prevents mislabelling and assures the correct label is placed on the correct feed;
- All deliveries of feeds, whether bagged or in bulk, shall be adequately labelled and contain appropriate instructions to assure the feed can be properly fed to the aquatic species intended; and
- Only tags for the product being bagged should be in the bagging area. Remaining or excess coded (dated) tags should be destroyed

immediately. For bulk feeds (as in large tonnages delivered by truck) the label and feeding instructions should be attached to the invoice or delivery documents.

Warehousing and Shipping

- Up to this point in feed production great care has been taken in the manufacturing and materials handling of feeds. Similar care must be taken in the warehousing and shipment of the final product.
- Sacked feeds must be stored in the warehouse off the ground on pallets away from sunlight with approximately one third of a meter between pallets to assure good air circulation.
- Storage should always be on a first-in, first-out basis.
- Storage of finished feeds must be carried out with the protection of the target species and human health as primary considerations. By meeting these objectives the feed miller should insure customer satisfaction.
- Shipping and distribution records should be maintained to facilitate recall of specific production batches/runs to the mill if and when an error occurs in processing.
- Bulk feed shipping documents should identify contents of each compartment in a truck or shipping container.
- All bagged products which are shipped should be in good condition (no ripped or otherwise leaking bags). All products sold and shipped should be properly weighed, and a copy of the shipping/billing order should accompany them.
- Bulk feed delivery trucks carrying medicated feeds should be appropriately flushed or sequenced, to assure that subsequent deliveries are not contaminated with unauthorised or detrimental chemicals, which could adversely affect other customers.

□□□

Chapter 25

Quality Control in Feed Manufacturing

Introduction

Quality control in the compound feed industry not only involves the verification of quality standards established for each feed ingredient as it is received into storage in the mill, but also involves the close monitoring of the quality of ingredients through the period of storage prior to usage and during its processing. Quality control continues as ingredients are merged during the mixing process and as they finally go into storage as compound feed.

Quality Control Procedures

Raw Materials

Feed manufacturing enterprises in developing countries operate under more difficult conditions than in developed countries. Problems of finance, management, and technical expertise aside, great difficulties in obtaining adequate supplies of raw materials are frequently encountered. Choices may also be restricted largely to feeds that are produced locally, since governments are reluctant to divert scarce foreign exchange for imports. Prices and availability of domestically produced feedstuffs are often subject to seasonal fluctuations while quality may also vary widely. Needed imports are made through agents with little experience in or responsibility for the quality of materials actually shipped. As a result, the need for quality control of both raw materials and finished products is greater for feed manufacturers in developing countries.

The purpose of quality control of raw materials is to ensure that minimum contract specifications are met. More precisely, it provides knowledge concerning the exact composition of raw materials and the levels of toxic substances normally present so that mixed feeds of the required nutritive value can be safely processed from them. These specifications are usually determined by a team consisting of the nutritionist, management personnel, and the quality control manager. The specifications relate to nutrient quality, cost, and the quality desired in the feedstuffs. Once the specifications are decided upon, they must be used and adhered to. Such a decision must be based on realistic reasoning, since it is useless to have specifications which are so narrow as to make purchasing impossible, or are so broad as to present severe problems for diet formulation.

Most contemporary feeds for livestock are formulated with the aid of a computer which calculates the cheapest product obtainable from available raw materials within constraints laid down for the nutritive value, toxicity, and palatability of the final product.

Preliminary Inspection

Materials received at the mill should be subjected to a thorough physical inspection to determine the following:

(a) Evidence of wetting - mould growth confirms water damage;

(b) Presence of scrap metals, stones, dirt, or other non-biological contaminants; and

(c) Presence of insects.

Moisture content of feed grains should be determined by one of the rapid procedures commercially available. Any consignment exceeding 13 percent moisture is especially prone to insect and mould attack and should be separated from other stored ingredients. Preferably, materials with high moisture content should not be taken into the store until after drying.

Sampling

Sampling is the most important activity in quality control, because no analysis can be better than the sample from which it is made. Hence, proper procedures for taking representative samples for quality evaluation are essential.

Sampling of bagged ingredients is done with a spear probe. The probe is inserted diagonally and as horizontally as possible, from one corner of the bag to the other. In lots of 1-10 bags, all bags are sampled. In larger lots, 10 percent of all bags are sampled. Materials received in bulk are sampled by using a scoop, according to the size of the consignment. For smaller than 10 t consignments, two samples per ton are taken. Larger consignments, up to 100 t, require one sample per ton or one sample for every two tons depending on the size of the consignment.

Samples taken in the above manner should be pooled, thoroughly mixed, and then reduced in size by quartering to between 1 and 2 kg in weight.

Oil cakes and other coarse materials are sampled by random selection of pieces from different parts of the entire consignment. Five pieces per ton of materials are considered sufficient. The pieces should then be ground, mixed thoroughly, and the sample reduced in size to between 1 and 2 kg as outlined above.

Samples submitted to the quality control laboratory should be placed in tightly sealed containers. Prior to chemical analysis, the samples must be reduced to a powder using a mortar.

Tests Required

For feedstuffs likely to contribute to both the protein and energy content of the final product, a "Weende" proximate analysis is usually conducted. This determines the moisture, crude protein, lipid, crude fibre, ash, and nitrogen-free extract content of the feedstuff.

Additional tests should be carried out on materials having a high ash content to determine the proportion of acid insoluble ash present, thus providing an indication of the amount of sand or other dirt present. This will also enable detection of any deliberate contamination of expensive feedstuffs such as fishmeal. Salt (NaCl) analysis of fish meal is also required for these same reasons, as well as to avoid excessive levels of sodium in the final diet.

Calcium and phosphorus determinations are routinely conducted on mineral feeds, such as bone meal, calcium phosphate and calcium carbonate sources. Other feedstuffs such as fish meal, and meat and bone meal are also analyzed for these two mineral elements.

Other Tests

The protein requirements of some cultured animal species are more exacting than others. For example, fish not only require higher protein levels in their diets but the protein quality requirements are also higher. The determination of amino acid content is a lengthy and complicated process requiring highly specialized, and expensive, equipment. However, it is advisable to test feedstuffs, such as fish meal, for lysine availability.

Certain feedstuffs contain natural toxins that, at high enough levels, are growth inhibitory and sometimes fatal to the animal consuming them. Principal among these are:

(a) *Urease*: An enzyme found in raw soybeans which produces toxicity through the hydrolysis of urea to toxic ammonia. The toasting process in soybean meal manufacture destroys the enzyme.

(b) *Gossypol*: An endogenous toxin present in the gland of cottonseed which persists during production of the meal unless removed by a special process, or, unless the cottonseed is a glandless variety.

(c) *Isothiocyanates*: cyanogenic glycosides are found in linseed and cassava. Much of the toxicity is eliminated during processing of the raw material.

(d) *Aflatoxin*: Aflatoxin is a class of extremely potent toxins produced by the mould Aspergillus flavus. Aflatoxin may be present in any materials produced and stored under hot and humid conditions and is usually found in groundnut cake, palm kernel cake, copra cake, and maize (which have not been properly dried after harvest).

Fats are rapidly oxidized in the warm tropics. Rancidity causes off-flavour in feeds. Levels of free fatty acids in expeller cakes, such as palm oil and copra cakes, have to be frequently checked. Unrefined palm oil or palm oil sludge, frequently used to increase the energy content of compounded feeds, contain high levels of free fatty acids.

Trace mineral and vitamin supplements form an important part of balanced diets for both poultry and livestock. The availability of these feed components from reliable sources makes it quite unnecessary to perform routine checks on their quality unless large volume purchases are involved. Sending samples to a reliable commercial laboratory obviates the great expenses of equipping a laboratory for such testing.

Finished Products

Quality control of the finished products consists of determining the manufacturing process to ensure that ingredients were added in the proportions required by the formulation. Inhomogeneity of the final product, due to improper mixing or unwanted ingredient separation, thus, can be detected. If it can be established that raw materials conform to specifications and that process control is adequate, then only periodic checks on the finished products are necessary.

Preliminary Inspection

Most modern mills are equipped with sieves and magnets along the material flow lines for removal of tramp metal, rocks, and other scrap contaminants. However, smaller operations may not have such features, and physical inspection of the finished product should be carried out to determine the presence of such contaminants. Any detection of foreign contaminants should be brought to the attention of the mill supervisor who could then determine if the contaminants originated in the raw material or if they were the result of improper maintenance within the mill premises.

Sampling

To detect product inhomogeneity and significant ingredient separation during the manufacturing process, sampling should be obtained during bagging-off time by taking a handful from every fifth bag of 40-50 bags and pooling the individual samplings. Testing for variability is best conducted by probing the bottom, middle, and top of a bag with a short probe. Tests may be made on each sample, or the samples from the same bags may be combined and mixed before analysis depending upon the question to be answered. The size of finished feed samples need only be half that required for raw materials, i.e., 0.5-1.0 kg after quartering. Samples submitted for chemical analysis should be placed in tightly sealed containers.

Tests Required

It is not uncommon for feed to be despatched to the customer on the same day it is manufactured, a day or two before chemical analysis on the product is completed. Therefore, one senses the importance of proper raw material quality control and the apparent irrelevance of quality testing on finished products. Nonetheless, quality control of finished products is necessary because it serves two important functions:

(a) It checks the manufacturing process, and

(b) It checks the quality specifications, or claims, established for the finished products.

If raw material quality control is properly conducted and if process control is adequate, then the only chemical tests required of finished products on a regular basis are for moisture and crude protein. Periodic inspections on other components of the "Weende" proximate analysis can also be scheduled.

Raw Material and Finished Product Storage

Both raw materials and finished feeds undergo deteriorative changes during storage. For raw materials, these changes represent a direct economic loss because of the resultant decrease in nutritive value. Finished products undergo changes which not only lower their nutritive value below minimum specifications but also affect their palatability and appearance.

Due to seasonal fluctuations in availability and price, it is often necessary to maintain large inventories of raw materials if demands are to be continuously satisfied at stable price levels. Six-month inventories of stocks of imported raw materials are not uncommon. In the tropics, such lengthy storage periods present special problems, because the two environmental factors which most affect deteriorative changes in stored feeds are temperature and relative humidity. The rates of chemical changes that normally occur are increased with increasing ambient temperatures. Insect and mould growth are also favoured by the warmer and more humid climate of the tropics. In addition, there is a distinct relationship between insect activity and chemical changes in stored feedstuffs. It is essential to keep them as cool and dry as possible) to minimize infestation by insect and rodent pests. Accordingly, warehouses should be constructed in such a way that the interior can be kept cool and dry with adequate ventilation to reduce micro-climatic variations created by the presence of the stored materials.

□□□

Chapter 26

Plant Cleanliness

General

The feed milling company should be committed to maintaining quality housekeeping programme that provides a safe and healthy environment for its employees and the community. The intent is to maintain mill properties in a manner that minimizes loss to persons or property and maximizes product quality assurance. Housekeeping is a direct responsibility of all employees, and each should be held accountable to do the things necessary to implement an effective housekeeping programme.

Practices

- Trash should be disposed of or recycled as appropriate.
- Feed and/or ingredient spills should be cleaned up immediately.
- Spilled materials should be put in designated, marked containers for proper disposal.

- Fugitive dust points should be investigated, evaluated, and corrective action taken.
- Offices and restrooms should be cleaned regularly.
- All employees should keep their work areas clean and orderly.
- All areas of the plant should be cleaned daily.
- Hand tools should be picked up and stored.
- Pallets of bagged products should be stacked neatly and in an orderly way.
- Broken bags should be taped and reclaimed as soon as possible.

Pest Control

- All broken windows should be repaired and the building kept tight to deny access to the mill from birds, rodents or other factors which may adversely affect the quality of the finished feed.
- Insects and rodents. The plant and warehouse should be baited and fogged as needed using approved pest control methods. Baits and fumigation should be done by trained personnel, preferably an approved, licensed pest control agency. A record should be kept of all pesticides used and the type of applications.

Chapter 27

Plant Maintenance and Repair

The plant maintenance program is vital to consistent production of high quality feeds and no less important to cost control and assurance to the customer that their feed will arrive on time and to formula specification. Equipment breakdowns are bad enough as they impede feed production, but at least as bad is machinery which is not working to design which may, through short weighing, or improper mixing, produce a defective feed. Such defective feed may, at the least, hurt the farmer's production and at worst create a serious failure. Also possible is a threat to human health. Keeping motors, scales, pellet dies, conveyors and all other components of the mill in proper working order is as important as formulation or the quality of ingredients which go into the finished feed. Mechanical or electronic failures may occur from time to time in a complex system like a feed mill, but proper attention to preventive maintenance will minimize down time and the prospect of the customer receiving feed which is out of specification. The latter may cause a costly recall of feed or possibly compensation for damages to the customer's crop, if the error is not found in a timely way. A good preventive maintenance programme should provide adequate maintenance at reasonable cost.

Preventive Maintenance Objectives

Reduce major repairs by correcting minor difficulties as soon as they are evident. This means listening to your operators who usually recognise before management that machinery is making a "funny noise" or other irregularity in performance of equipment. Maintain equipment in a more productive state. Keep it clean; repair or replace lost or worn parts immediately. Follow the machinery manual recommendations. Improve scheduling of repairs. Do not postpone needed repairs. Delaying repairs usually results in much more costly problems later on.

Maintain safety: Some parts as they become worn become dangerous, as in worn chain or belt drives. Staffs are valuable and injuries are costly from the standpoint of lost time and training replacements, not to mention adverse impacts on employee morale.

Improved customer service: A well-maintained mill looks good to the customer and helps assure the customer that the feed is made correctly the first time.

Reduce overall operating costs: The miller of aquaculture feeds benefits from a well maintained facility through reduced costs of operation and customer satisfaction.

Provide trained maintenance personnel: Training of maintenance staff should be a high priority with high-level management oversight. Too often maintenance is seen as the bottom of the ladder, when in reality the quality and training of staff for this important responsibility should be paramount.

Building and Grounds Maintenance

- The building grounds shall be adequately drained and maintained to be reasonably free from litter, waste, refuse, uncut weeds or grass, standing water and improperly stored equipment.
- The buildings shall be maintained in a reasonably clean and orderly manner.
- Adequate space, ventilation and lighting shall be maintained for the proper performance of all manufacturing, storing, labelling,

quality assurance and maintenance aspects of feed manufacturing.

Preventive Maintenance Areas

- A checklist is required to highlight generalised preventive maintenance functions, which are to be checked periodically. Each plant manager should take this guideline and revise it to conform to the actual conditions of his plant.
- A log (record) book or computer record should be maintained on a daily basis. Careful attention should be paid to the equipment manufacturer's suggested maintenance schedule(s).

❑❑❑

Chapter 28

Economics in Preparation of Turkey Feed

Turkey farming is gaining popularity in Tamil Nadu. Turkey farming can be practiced in an integrated manner by a combination of certain other activities like feed mixing along with it. To perform an activity efficiently, all the raw materials has to be made available in the given area. In the last decade or so, turkey farming faced innumerous problems especially due to the high mortality of turkey poults. But of late, the problem has been solved to a large extend due to scientific rearing methods. Therefore turkey feed mixing unit can be started, in areas where turkey farms are concentrated. Turkey farming can be carried out as a commercial enterprise rather than as backyard.

Feed mixing unit can be started to supply the required feed to the turkey units. The feed prepared can range from 100 kg to 2 tonnes a day. The feed mill can also cater to the needs of other livestock. Feed can be supplied to calves, cow, buffalo, horse, sheep and goat and poultry species like chicken, turkey, guinea fowl, geese, emu and ostrich. The feed mill has to be installed according to the market requirement.

Economics of a 250 kg/day capacity feed unit :

Requirements:		
Grinding unit	-	100 sq.ft.
Mixing unit	-	100 sq.ft.
Feed ingredients and equipments:		
Godown	-	100 sq.ft.
Machines	-	1.5 Hp pulveriser
If necessary a 250 kg capac ity feed mixer		
Weighing machine(250 kg)	-	1
Hand mixer	-	1
I.Non-Recurring Expenditure		
1. Building (200 Rs / sq.feet.) for 300 sq.ft	-	Rs.60,000
2. 1.5 Hp pulveriser (capacity 25kg/hour)	-	Rs.13,000
Electric supply accessories	-	Rs.500
Weighing machine	-	Rs.1000
Miscellaneous cost	-	Rs.500
Total		**Rs.75,000**
II. Recurring expenditures:		
1.Feed ingredients required to prepare 250 kg of mash	-	Rs.2775
2.Electricity cost	-	Rs.50
3. Cost of gunny bags at Rs.10 per gunny bag.	-	Rs.50
Depreciation for non-recurring expenditure (10%)	-	Rs.21
Interest for non recurring expenditures (12%)	-	Rs.26
Total		**Rs.2922**
III. Profit:		
Cost of 250 kg turkey pre brooder feed at Rs. 13/kg.	-	Rs.3,250
Profit percentage per day	-	Rs.3250-2922 = Rs.228
Profitpercentage per month	-	Rs.228 x 30 = Rs. 6840
Profit percentage per year	-	Rs. 6840 x 12 = Rs. 82080

I. Feed Unit of 250 kg/day Capacity

This is suitable for a small scale feed unit. This can be installed in villages to supply feed for the local market area. The aim of the feed mill has to be to supply feed to all the livestock in the nearby area There has to be a scope for marketing at least 250 kg feed for the enterprise to be profitable.

II. 2 Tonnes/day Capacity Feed Mill

In this type of feed unit, a hammer mill has to be combined with a mixer. As far as possible, it is better to have a four wheeler to transport

Economics of a 2 tonnes/day capacity feed unit

I.Non-Recurring Expenditure		
1. Building	-	
To install machines		1000 sq.ft.
To store feed ingredients	-	1000 sq.ft.
Cost for building(200 Rs / sq.feet. for 2000 sq.feet	-	Rs.4,00,000
2.hammer mill(17 inch) with 10 Hp motor	-	Rs.50,000
Electrical weighing machine	-	Rs.10000
Machine for stitching gunny bags	-	Rs.5000
Electric supply accessories	-	Rs.5000
Miscellaneous cost	-	Rs.5000
Total		Rs.5,45,500
II. Recurring expenditures:		
1.Feed ingredients required to prepare 2 tonnes of mash	-	Rs.20,000
2.Electricity cost per day	-	Rs.500
3. Labours - 2 Rs.100 per labour	-	Rs.200
3. Cost of 40 gunny bags at Rs.10 p er gunny bag.	-	Rs.400
Depreciation for non-recurring expenditure (10%)	-	Rs.21
Interest for non recurring expenditures (12%)	-	Rs.26
Total		**Rs.21428**
III. Profit:		
Cost of 2000 kg turkey pre brooder feed at Rs. 13/kg.	-	Rs.26,000
Profit per day	-	Rs. 26,000 - 21,428 = Rs.4572
Profit per month	-	Rs.4572 x 30 = Rs. 1,37,160
Profit per year	-	Rs. 16,45,920

feed and feed ingredients. This not only increases the efficiency of the feed mill but also saves time. To install this feed mill, it is necessary to have three phase electric power. The hammer mill and mixer used in this feed mill need to have a capacity to handle 250 kg feed per hour.

III. Economics of a Feed Mill (4,500 tonnes per annum -Installed Capacity)

Technical Assumptions

a) The unit proposes to work at least 300 days per annum on single shift basis.

b) The unit can achieve its full capacity utilization during the 2nd year of operation.

c) The wages for skilled workers is taken as per prevailing rates in this type of industry.

d) Interest rate for total capital investment is calculated @ 12% per annum.

e) The entrepreneur is expected to raise 20-25% of the capital as margin money.

f) The unit proposes to construct own building.

g) Costs of machinery and equipment are based on average prices enquired from machinery manufacturers.

Implementation Schedule

Project implementation will take a period of 8 months. Break-up of the activities and relative time for each activity is shown below:

Scheme preparation and approval	:	01 month
SSI provisional registration	:	1-2 months
Sanction of financial supports etc.	:	2-5 months
Installation of machinery and power connection	:	6-8 months
Trial run and production	:	01 month

Technical Aspects

Location

The unit can be set up in any rural and semi-urban area where the raw material is available in plenty and local demand exists for the product. The availability of water, power, and road connectivity are also to be considered while selecting the location.

Process of Manufacture

The animal feed comprises of various formulations such as poultry feed and cattle feed to meet the requirements of chicken, turkey, milch cattle etc.

Pollution Control

There is no major pollution problem associated with this industry except for disposal of waste which should be managed appropriately. The entrepreneurs are advised to take "No Objection Certificate" from the State Pollution Control Board.

Energy Conservation

Adequate care should be to minimise the wastage of electric power.

Production Capacity

Quantity	:	1,000 tpa
Installed capacity	:	4.5 00 tpa
Optimum capacity utilization	:	70%
Working days	:	300/annum
Manpower	:	18
Utilities		
Motive Power	:	20 kW
Water	:	5 kL/day

Financial Aspects

Fixed Capital

Land & Building	**:**	**Amount (Rs. lakh)**
Land 1000 sq.m.	:	1.25
Built up Area 250 sq. m..	:	8.25
Total cost of Land and Building	:	9.50

Machinery and Equipment

Description	**Amount (Rs. lakh)**
Screw conveyor, single deck vibroscreen, bucket elevator, hammer mill, suction blower, batch mixer, peddle conveyor, molasses and mixer, bucket elevator, bagging and conveying system, aspirators, electrical control panel	12.00
Erection and electrification @ 10% of machinery cost	1.20
Office furnitre & fixtures	0.40
Total	**13.60**

Pre-operative Expenses

Consultancy fee, project report, deposits with electricity department etc.	0.5

Total Fixed Capital

(5.1.1+5.1.2+5.1.3)	22.00

Recurring Expenses Per Annum

Personnel

Designation	No.	Salary Per month	Amount (Rs.lakh)
Factory Manager/Entrepreneur	1	8000	0.96
Supervisor	1	5000	0.60
Skilled worker	2	2500	0.60
Unskilled workers(8 months)	14	2000	3.36
			5.52
Perquisites @15%			0.83
Total	**18**		**6.35**

Raw Material Including Packaging Materials

Particulars	Qty.(MT)	Rate/MT	Amount (Rs. lakh)
Broken rice, maize, rice bran, Fish meal etc.	1150	3250	37.38
Gunny bags	10,500 No.	12 each	01.22
Total			**38.60**

Utilities	Amount (Rs. lakh)
Power	0.58
Water	0.02
Total	**0.60**

Other Contingent Expenses	Amount (Rs. lakh)
Repairs and maintenance@10% Consumables & spares	1.32
Transport & Travel	0.60
Publicity	
Postage & stationery	
Telephone	
Insurance	0.18
Total	**2.10**

Total Recurring Expenditure	Amount (Rs. lakh)
(5.2.1+ 5.2.2+ 5.2.3+ 5.2.4)	47.65

Working Capital

Recurring Expenditure for 3 months	12.00

Total Capital Investment	Amount (Rs. lakh)
Fixed capital (Refer 5.1.4)	22.00
Working capital (Refer 5.3)	12.00
Total	**34.00**

Financial Analysis

Cost of Production (per annum)	Amount (Rs. lakh)
Recurring expenses (Refer 5 .2.5)	47.65
Depreciation on building @5%	0.41
Depreciation on machinery @10%	1.32
Depreciation on furniture @20%	0.08
Interest on Capital Investment @12%	4.04
Total	**53.50**

Sale Proceeds (Turnover) per year

Item	Qty. (MT)	Rate (MT)	Amount (Rs.lakh)
Feed (assorted)	1,000	6800	68.00

Net Profit per year

=	Sales – Cost of production
=	68.00 – 53.50
=	Rs. 14.50 lakh

Net Profit Ratio

$$= \frac{\text{Net profit X 100}}{\text{Sales}}$$

$$= \frac{14.50 \text{ X } 100}{68}$$

$$= 21.30\%$$

Rate of Return on Investment

$$= \frac{\text{Net profit X 100}}{\text{Capital Investment}}$$

$$= \frac{14.50 \text{ X } 100}{34}$$

$$= 42.60\%$$

Annual Fixed Cost

	Amount (Rs. Lakh)
All depreciation	1.81
Interest	4.04
40% of salary, wages, utility, contingency	3.62
Insurance	0.18
Total	**9.65**

Break Even Point

$$= \frac{\text{Annual Fixed Cost X 100}}{\text{Annual Fixed Cost + Profit}}$$

$$= \frac{9.65 \text{ X } 100}{9.65 + 14.50}$$

$$= 40\%$$

□□□

are [illegible]
involv[illegible]
the tr[illegible] periods pose [illegible] problems,
because [illegible] environmental factors which most affect deteriorative
changes in [illegible] feeds are temperature and relative humidity. The
rates of chemical changes that normally occur are increased with
increasing ambient temperatures. Insect and mould growth are also
favoured by the warmer and more humid climate of the tropics. In
addition, there is a distinct relationship between insect activity and
chemical changes in stored feedstuffs. It is essential to keep them as
cool and dry as possible) to minimize infestation by insect and rodent
pests. Accordingly, warehouses should be constructed in such a way
that the interior can be kept cool and dry with adequate ventilation to
reduce micro-climatic variations created by the presence of the stored
materials.

Chapter 29

Draft Code of Practice for Good Animal Feeding (FAO, 1998)

Introduction

This code of practice applies to feed manufacturing and to the use of all feeds, other than those consumed while grazing free range. The objective of the code is to encourage adherence to Good Manufacturing Practice (GMP) during the procurement, handling, storage, processing (however minimal), and distribution of feed for food producing animals. A further objective is to encourage good feeding practices on the farm. There are potential risks to human health associated with the contamination of feed with chemical or biological agents. This code outlines the means by which these hazards can be controlled by adopting appropriate processing, handling and monitoring procedures. The principle approaches required for assessing food borne hazards to human health have been outlined elsewhere.

General Management

The ultimate responsibility for the production of safe and wholesome feed lies with the producer or manufacturer who should produce feeds with as low a level of hazard as possible and comply with any applicable statutory requirements. The effective implementation of GMP protocols will ensure that:

- Buildings and equipment, including processing machinery, will be constructed in a manner which permits ease of operation, maintenance and cleaning;
- Staff will be adequately trained and that training is kept up to date;
- Records will be maintained concerning source of ingredients, formulations including details and source of all additives, date of manufacture, processing conditions and any date of dispatch,
- Details of any transport and destination;
- Water used in feed manufacture is of potable quality;
- Machinery coming into contact with feed is dried following any wet cleaning process;
- Condensation is minimised; sewage, waste and rain water is disposed of in a manner that
- Ensures that equipment, ingredients and feed are not contaminated; and
- Feed processing plants, storage facilities and their immediate surroundings are kept clean and free of pests.

Raw Materials of Animal and Plant Origin

Raw materials of animal and plant origin should be obtained from reputable sources, preferably with a supplier warranty. Monitoring of ingredients should include inspection and sampling of ingredients for contaminants using risk based protocols. Laboratory testing, where undertaken, should be by standard methods. Ingredients should meet acceptable, and if applicable, statutory standards for levels of pathogens, mycotoxins, herbicides, pesticides and other contaminants which may give rise to human health hazards. In order to control the spread of specific pathogens it may be necessary to specify, for any given ingredient, the country and species of origin and any treatment process used prior to purchase. Care should be taken to preserve the identity of such material after procurement to facilitate any tracking that might be required.

Minerals, Supplements, Veterinary Drugs and Other Additives

Minerals, supplements, veterinary drugs and other additives should be obtained from reputable manufacturers who guarantee the concentration and purity of ingredients and provide instructions for correct use.

General Management of Feeds

Feeds should be stored so as to prevent deterioration and contamination. Processed feeds should be separated from unprocessed ingredients. Containers and equipment used for transport, storage, conveying, handling and weighing should be kept clean. Equipment should be ?flushed' with ?clean' feed material between batches of different formulations to control cross contamination. Pathogen control procedures, such as pasteurization or the addition of an organic acid to inhibit mould growth, should be used where appropriate and results monitored. Apart from feeds fed moist, such as silage and by-products of brewing, ingredients and feeds should be kept dry to limit fungal and bacterial growth. This may necessitate ventilation and temperature control.

□□□

Chapter 30

Structure of Egg and Its Parts

Egg is an important nutritious food for human being. It is consumed all over the world. Egg is one of the food where adulteration is not possible. Fertile egg is used for hatching. The nutrition required for the growth of embryo is completely supplied by the egg itself.

Shape of egg

Egg is oval in shape. One end of the egg is broad and flat and the other end is narrow. The diameter of the broader end is large. This shape of the egg is very important for hatching of poults.

Parts of egg

- Shell
- Shell membrane
- Albumen
- Yolk

Shell

The eggshell is made up of 93-98% of calcium carbonate. More than 8000 small pores are present on the eggshell. The exchange of oxygen and carbon dioxide takes place through these pores. Compared to the other parts of egg, more number of pores are seen in the broader end of the egg.

Shell Membrane

There are two membranes beneath the eggshell. The outer shell membrane is seen below the shell. The inner shell membrane closely surrounds the albumen. The outer membrane is three times thicker than the inner membrane. These two membranes are firmly attached to the shell.

At the broader end, these two membranes are separated by a space called air cell. In newly laid eggs, the depth of egg shell will be only 3mm, if the eggs are stored for a longer time its moisture gets reduced and the depth of air cell increases up to 8mm. Thus the period of egg storage can be identified by the measurement of air cell depth.

Albumen

It consists of 4 layers, namely, inner thick albumen, inner thin albumen, outer thick albumen, and outer thin albumen. The inner thick layer is very close to the yolk immediately surrounding the vitelline membrane of the yolk. The thick albumen twists into two chords on either sides of the yolk called chalazae.

Functions of Chalazae

It provides warmth to the developing embryo. It also holds the yolk firmly in its central position and serves as an anchor for yolk Albumen not only provides nutrition to the developing embryo but also protects it against the adverse environment.

Egg Yolk

Yolk is formed in ovary itself. The vitelline membrane surrounds it. Yolk consists of concentric layer of lighter and darker yolk materials. The lighter yolk material, which joins the germ spot is the latebrae. The nutrition needed for the growth of embryo is found in the yolk itself. It consists of 48% water and 32.5% fat. Protein, vitamins, minerals and cholesterol are also present in the yolk.

Germ Spot

Germ spot is the reproductive cell. It is a lighter coloured spot located on the surface of yolk, just under the vitelline membrane. When the egg is poured on a plate, the germ spot is easily seen as a small white spot. In a fertile egg the germ spot is larger when compared to the germ spot in an infertile egg. This is called as blastodisc. The growth of embryo starts from this disc.

Parts of an egg and its composition

Parts of an egg	Percentage	Water%	Protein%	Fat%	Ash%
Egg	100	65.5	11.8	11.0	11.7
Albumen	58	88.0	11.0	0.2	0.8
Yolk	31	48	17.5	32.5	2.0
Egg shell	11	-	-	-	100

Development of Egg

Reproductive System

a) Male Reproductive System

In tom turkey, sperms are produced in the testes. The testes are paired, small ovoid structure lying on the dorsal body wall, on either side of vertebral column and anterior to the kidney. From the testes the sperms are transported to the cloaca by means of vas deferens.

b) Female Reproductive System

It consists of two ovaries and two oviducts, but out of two only the left ovary and oviduct is functional at time of hatching, while the right ovary is atrophied.

Ovary

The ovary is responsible for the formation of yolk. In a single female turkey around 900-3600 over are seen.

Oviduct

The oviduct is a long highly coiled tube. Oviduct extends from the ovary to the cloaca. It has five different parts namely infundibulum, magnum, isthmus, uterus and vagina.

Uses of different parts of oviduct

Parts	Time taken for the formation of egg	Formation of egg
Infundibulum	20 minutes	Capture of ova After the complete development, the yolk comes out of the follicle and enters the infundibulum. If the egg does not reach the infudibulum, it falls into the lower abdomen and get absorbed
Magnum	3 hours	Albumen formation Dense white albumen is secreted in the magnum. After that it surrounds the yolk. Chalazae formation Even though the chalazae is developed in the magnum itself it can be seen only when it reaches the uterus.
Isthmus	11/4 hours	Shell membrane formation Both the outer and inner membranes are formed in the isthmus
Uterus	18 to 20 hours	Egg shell formation Eggshell is formed in the uterus. Around 3 grams of calcium is required for the formation of eggshell. The development of shell process is very slow during the first 3 hours but it increases in the next 5 hours.
Vagina		Egg laying ovi position After the full development, the egg reaches the cloaca. Before it goes to the cloaca, it gets rotated at 180° angle so that the broader end comes out first.

Fertility and hatchability

The egg, which is produced without the act of mating, is called as table egg. Egg laid by hen turkey after mating with the tom turkey is used for hatching. It is called as fertile egg. Turkey egg's fertility, hatching ability and quality of turkey poult depends on the environment and its genetic makeup, the age of turkey hen, its nutritional status, diseases resistance and environmental factors.

Fertile egg are obtained from the superior turkey tom and hen turkey at ratio of 1: 4. The fertile egg is obtained only after 4 days of mating. The fertility may get reduced after 4 or 5 days of removal of the tom turkey. Even though the tom turkey is removed female lays fertile egg because of its ability to store the sperms within it. The fertility and hatching ability of egg decreases with increase in age of the bird.

□□□

Chapter 31

Embryonic Development

The developmental changes that take place from the time of fertilization of gametes to hatching of the poults are given below in this chapter.

Fertilization of Gametes

Blastodisc seen in the yolk unites with the male sperm which is called fertilization of gametes. This takes place in infundibulum and magnum junction. This is the first step in the embryonic development.

Developmental Changes Taking Place before the Egg is Laid

After the fertilization, egg with the single cell under goes cell division and develops into single layer (32 cells) epiblast. After that, cells undergo second cell division and develops into two layers hypoblast which seen below the epiblast. Blastoderm in the egg divides when it passes through the oviduct. At same time when it passes through the magnum different layers of albumen is formed and it surrounds the yolk. This albumen provides nutrition and immunity to the developing embryo. Finally the eggshell is formed when it reaches the uterus.

In egg, embryo is around 4mm in size as a small white colour disc. After the egg is laid, it is kept in the chiller room. The temperature of the room should be 65°F (18.3°C). At this temperature growth of embryo is arrested.

Changes Taking Place after the Egg is Laid

During first 24 hours of incubation, a small streak like structure develops in the embryo is called as primordial streak. After the next 18 hours more structures develop from this streak.

Between epiblast and hypoblast, epiblastic cells changes into coil like structure and develops into a third layer called mesoderm. Most of the body parts develop from these three layers. They are as follows:

Layers	Body parts
Ectoderm	Skin, wings, beak, nervous system, claws, eye lens, retina, digestive system
Mesoderm	Bones, muscles, circulatory, excretory, and reproductive system.
Endoderm	Respiratory and endocrine system

Embryonic Membranes

Yolk layer, amnion, chorion and allantois are layers necessary for the growth of embryo. The yolk layer is seen surrounding the yolk. This layer is highly vascularised. After hatching, this layer may develop into a small air filled structure which is seen adjacent to the intestine. Through this structure, nutrition is absorbed directly into the blood vessels.

Amnion

Develops within 2 to 3 days of incubation. The amniotic fluid is formed as soon as the amnion is formed. This fluid protects the embryo from the water loss, heat stress and any shock from the environment.

Chorion

Develops once the amniotic layer is formed. Chorion gets connected with white albumen. When the albumen is completely used this layer gets united with the allantois.

Allantois

Develops from the intestine of embryo and it is seen between the amnion and chorion. Chorionic layer unites with allantois and form chorio-allantoic layer. This layer is highly vascularised. Until the lung develops in the embryo, exchange of gas takes place through this layer. This layer also helps in the transfer of calcium from the shell to the embryo. By this, the eggshell becomes week and this helps the poult at the time of hatching. The urates which is formed in the kidney of embryo is excreted in the amniotic fluid.

Body Parts Development

First 1-2 days

Less than 1 cm, a small white coloured flat disc is seen on the yolk. The white albumen is seen just like a mist without any blood vessels.

3-9 days

The yolk is highly vascularised. The leg and beak develops but the small dot seen over the beak is absent.

10-15 days

First the feathers are formed. Then the nostril over the beak is formed.

16-24 days

The layer surrounding the yolk gets absorbed and the shape necessary for the hatching is achieved.

25-27 days

Yolk layer is completely absorbed. Pipping of eggshell and hatching of chicks take place.

Position of Embryo for Hatching

Muscular movements are first step in hatching. Movement of muscular parts in the embryonic neck and back pushes the head front. Through this the broader end comes in upward direction. After that yolk layer get absorbed into the embryo. Finally the allantoic layer gets teared and this layer gets separated from the air cell. The level of carbon dioxide in the embryo's blood induces the pulmonary respiration. If the position of poult is correct, then the beak of turkey will pierce the air cell. Within the next 5 or 6 hours the eggshell gets broken. Blood flows in chorio allantoic layer get reduced when pulmonary respiration starts. Thus only small amount of blood loss occurs, if this layer is ruptured. Even though the pulmonary respiration takes place, exchange of gas through the chorio allantoic layer will continue. But 1 or 2 hours before hatching this get reduced and respiration takes place through the lungs.

Breaking of Eggshell

Once the respiration through the lungs gets started, the turkey poult breaks the eggshell from the right side to left side and comes out. This takes about 30 minutes to 2 hours.

□□□

Chapter 32

Factors Required for Incubation

Main factors for hatching of eggs in artificial incubation method are providing appropriate temperature, air humidity, ventilation and turning of eggs.

Temperature

If the temperature is higher, then growth of embryo and its respiration rate gets increased as a result more amount of carbon dioxide is released. And also, embryo grows in sideward direction and this leads to the death of embryo. If the temperature is lower, the growth and respiration is restricted and embryo dies.

Temperature Required for Incubation

Incubation (weeks)	Temperature (°F)	
	Lower level	Higher level
1	99.5	101.0
2	99.5	100.0
3	99.0	101.0
4	99.0	101.0

Humidity

In setter 11-12% of its total weight is lost while in hatchery 3-4% of its total weight is lost. In the initial stage of incubation if there is more loss of moisture, then embryo gets attached to egg shell and dies. In the egg, vaporization of moisture depend on temperature, speed of air, size of egg and thickness of eggshell in the incubator. At particular temperature the humidity of air, expressed in percentage is called as relative humidity. This can be measured using wet and dry bulb thermometer.

In setter, up to 24 days the relative humidity should be 65%. In Hatcher for next 4 days it should be 70-75%. The wet bulb thermometer reading changes on basis of movement of air. So the humidity cannot be measured in incubator when there is no movement of air. In large incubator the temperature, speed of air and humidity is related to each other. At time of hatching the temperature will be reduced and humidity will be at higher side.

Way to Increase the Humidity

- By changing the water plates in incubator the humidity can be increased.
- By using absorbing cotton in water plate the vaporization can be increased leading to increase in humidity.
- By using more water plates in the incubator with no circulating fans, the humidity can be increased.
- By sprinkling water over the air circulating pores, humidity can be increased.

If the humidity is at higher side the embryo inside the shell dies. If the humidity is at lower side then the moisture in the egg becomes vaporized, and the poults get attached to the eggshell. Sometime if it hatches, the chicks will be small & slender and crawling of poults will be noticed.

Relative Humidity Level

Wet thermometer level (°F)	98	99	100	101 (°F)
	Dry thermometer level Relative humidity percentage			
90	72	70	68	65
89	70	67	65	63
88	67	65	63	60
87	65	62	60	57
86	61	39	57	54
85	58	56	54	59
84	55	53	51	49
83	53	51	48	46
82	50	48	46	44
81	48	45	43	41
80	45	43	41	39

Ventilation

For hatching of egg, 24% of oxygen is required. The level of carbon dioxide should not exceed more than 0.5%. And also, in incubator, for 1000 turkey eggs the flow of air should be 100 cubic feet per minute. If the flow of air is not regular, then hatching of poult is affected. It leads to the death of embryo inside the egg itself. In such embryo following condition are seen:

1. Only 19-20 days growth of embryo is noticed
2. It is not dry

More than 8000 pores are seen in the eggshell, through which the exchange of oxygen and carbon dioxide take place. Initial stage of embryonic development the lungs will be under developed, so for first 5 days respiration take place through the blood circulation in the vitelline membrane. The air to reach the blood circulation has to pass through the pores in eggshell and white albumen. In embryo, the allantois is formed, after 4 or 5 days. This layer is seen very close to the eggshell. Thus allantois functions as first respiratory organ. After the hatching the lungs acts as respiratory organ. So at the time of embryonic development enough air should be there in incubator.

Factors that Affect the Ventilation

1. Temperature and humidity in the incubator.
2. Number of eggs in the incubator.

3. Incubation period.
4. Speed of air inside incubator.

Turning of Egg

At time of incubation the turkey will turn its egg naturally. In artificial method of hatching the turning of eggs should be done.

Importance of Turning of Eggs

This is done to prevent the attachment of the embryo to the shell membrane and also to supply nutrition to the embryo.

In white albumen fat is totally absent. So its specific gravity is similar to the specific gravity of water. But fat content is higher in egg yolk. So its specific gravity will be less than the water. So the yolk floats in the albumen and also developing embryo will be seen in the upper portion of egg yolk. If turning is not done then yolk will pass through albumen and come close to the eggshell. Thus embryo is trapped between the yolk and eggshell, so it is not able to use the nutrition and leads to the death of embryo. As embryo is close to the shell organisms easily infect it. So turning should be done regularly for the proper growth of embryo. In natural method of incubation, by means of turning the temperature required for its growth is easily acquired from its mother.

During the last 3 days of incubation turning of eggs should not be done. This is because poults reach the position of hatching and also of embryo will be larger in size by the last 3 or 4 days. So by this time most of the egg yolk will be utilized for the development and so there is no chance for the death of embryo.

In commercial hatcheries, the turning of eggs is done fully by automatic machine for every one hour. The angle of turning of eggs should be 45^0.

□□□

Chapter 33

Selection of Eggs for Hatching

In turkey farming hatchery is an important division. Hence selection of eggs for hatching should be done carefully. If the selected egg has any defects then its hatching ability is affected. The egg selected for hatching usually has 15 reasons for their defects. The reasons for their defects are given below.

In the farm, due to unavoidable circumstances, the eggs for hatching may become dirty or cracks or break in eggshell is seen. To avoid this, proper facilities for the egg laying should be provided. The litter material should be changed frequently. Proper handling of the eggs should be done. Do not allow the turkey to lay the eggs on floor or wooden board.

Biological Causes

The body temperature of turkey is important factor that affect the quality of eggs. If body temperature is high then the egg shell gets affected and leads to thin shell. And also environment and genetic defect is also an important factor in affecting the quality of egg. If the egg is seen in the uterus for prolonged period then there are changes for following defects. They are as follows :

- Different shapes of eggs
- More calcium deposit in eggshell.

Eggs with more calcium deposits should not be kept for incubation. Because high calcium deposits will close the egg pores and hence the exchange of gases does not take place leading to death of embryo.

Collection of Eggs for Incubation

The eggs should be collected periodically. Mostly 70% of eggs are laid only in the afternoon. The eggs should be cleaned and then incubated.

Following qualities are required for selection of hatching eggs:

Weight of Egg

Average weight of turkey egg is 70-75g. If the eggs which are large or small it should not be used for hatching.

Shape of Egg

The selected egg should be oval in shape. If the shape is irregular hatching does not take place properly.

Quality of Eggshell

Cracked eggshell, thin-shelled eggs and shell with more pores should not be selected. Similarly dirty eggs should not be selected. Because the dirt in the eggs may block the small pores, so the exchange of gas does not take place and leads to the death of embryo. And also dirt in eggs leads to spread of infection to the embryo, so only clean egg should be used.

Quality of Inner Parts of Eggs

By means of candling the growth of embryo should be checked. If the proper growth is not seen then such type of eggs should be removed. Similarly the ratio of white and yellow part should be only 2:1.

Inbreeding

Hatching ability of eggs collected from the inbreed turkey will be lesser.

Protection of Eggs from Entry of Organism

Naturally the entry of the organisms through the eggs is prevented. More than 8000 small pores are seen in eggshell. Most of the pores' size will be smaller than the size of organisms so their entry is restricted. But some pores will be larger in size so the organisms enter easily. It depends on two major reasons :

They are :

- Thickness of the eggshell
- Quality of eggshell

The cuticle seen over the eggshell naturally prevents the entry of microorganisms. The inner and outer shell membrane also acts as a barrier. The higher level of acid content in the white albumen will prevent the growth of organisms; similarly the vitelline membrane in the egg yolk protects the growing embryo from organisms.

Cleaning of Eggs

Cleaning of hatching eggs is very important because within 30 minutes the organisms can easily enter the shell.

Fumigation

Practically, eggs are fumigated with formaldehyde gas or ozone gas.

Ultraviolet Rays

This type of cleaning is done only in large-scale commercial farms.

Disinfection

The disinfectant is mixed with the luke warm water and this can be used to clean the eggs.

Storage of Eggs

In most of commercial hatchery farm, before keeping the eggs in incubator, it should be kept in the cold storage room for 2 to 7 days. Turkey's eggs should not be kept in the storage room for more than two weeks. Keeping the eggs in cold storage room restricts the growth of embryo.

Cold Storage Room

After cleaning the eggs, it should be kept in the cold storage room. It takes one day for complete chilling of eggs. The temperature of room should 57-59^{0}F. If the egg is kept for more than 10 days then the temperature should be reduced to 54-55^{0}F. The relative humidity should be 70-80%.

If the egg is kept in storage room for more than 10 days then following steps should be done to increasing its hatching ability.

- Wrap the egg in plastic cover.
- Turning of eggs should be done at least 3 times a day.
- The narrow end of egg should be kept in downward direction.
- The temperature and relative humidity of room should be recorded twice a day.
- The eggs should be kept in incubator based on its egg laying. The older eggs should be kept for incubation first followed by new eggs.

Effects of Storage of Eggs

The incubation period of egg is extended, if it is kept in cold storage room. Storage of eggs for one day will extend its incubation period for one hour.

The hatching ability is reduced if the eggs are stored for long time. Storing the eggs for more than 6 days, will reduce the hatching ability to 0.5-1.5% for each day.

If the egg is stored for more than 14 days then the quality of chicks are affected and similarly the weight of chicks will be reduced.

❑❑❑

Chapter 34

Incubation

The incubation period for the different avian species is

Breeds	Incubation period (days)
Chicken	21
Turkey	28
Duck	28
Swan	33-35
Goose	29-31
Guinea fowl	26-28
Pigeon	16-18
White quail	23
Japanese quail	17-18
Ostrich	42
Emu	54
Peacock	28

Hatching of eggs in natural method

If number of eggs kept for hatching is less, then hen turkey/chicken is used.

Hatching of eggs in artificial method

If more eggs are hatched at a time, then artificial method is used. About 2000 years before, the Chinese and Egyptians used artificial method for hatching.

Modern instruments

In 1749, a Physics scientist namely, Rhimer used the machine for hatching in which the temperature was controlled. In 1770, John Cambian, used fires from the broilers for hatching of eggs. The capacity of it was 20,000 eggs. In 1922, Peter Syam, an American invented the incubator which works in electricity. There are three types of incubator. They are,

- Still air
- Cabinet type
- Walk in or drive in type.

Basically in any type of incubator, the door, which does not conduct heat, is used. Its inner temperature is kept controlled. In the entire incubator a panel is seen through which working of machine can be seen.

Points to be remember before buying an incubator

- Capacity of incubator
- The availability, price of spare parts and its quality

Still air incubator (without inner air circulation)

In this type of incubator, fewer number of eggs are kept for incubation. Its capacity is 10 to 100 eggs. In this circulating fans and automatic turning of eggs are not provided. In this incubator, heat is produced by using electricity, paddy straw, paddy husk, kerosene, and biogas. The temperature of incubator should be 102-103°F. The temperature is higher because of absence of inner air circulation.

The humidity is 60-70%. This humidity is obtained by keeping the eggs in one rack and other rack filled with water which is kept below that. Water used for incubation should be clean because the dirt in the water prevents the vaporization of water and thus relative humidity will be reduced.

The eggs are turned at an angle of 45° and it is turned at the rate of 4-6 times per day. This type of incubator has only one rack and there is no air circulation, so the eggs can be set only once. After 7 days the candling of all eggs should be done and the infertile eggs should be removed.

Cabinet type of incubator

Difference between the cabinet and space air are as follows:

- In this eggs are kept vertically with broader end in upward direction and narrower end in downward direction.
- The inner air circulation is controlled by means of electric fans or stirrer.
- Capacity of eggs is more than 1000

Multi deck cabinet type

This type of incubator should be functioning continuously. In this, eggs have to be kept in setter for one or two times in week and then transferred to hatcher. In this more number of eggs can be kept in space. These incubators are electrically controlled. The temperature is produced by means of electricity. To produce the requires temperature, coiled electric wires are kept inside. To keep the temperature at optimum level thermostats are used. The fan that is kept inside is used for air circulation and for spreading the temperature. Turning is done automatically. In old cabinet type the setter and hatcher are kept in the same instrument. But nowadays setter and hatcher are kept separately.

In this type the setter room is larger. One fourth of total eggs are kept in the rack for once in a week. While keeping the eggs for easy identification each rack should be coloured differently or bit of paper should be used. The red, white and blue are the commonly used colours. This helps in easy transfer of eggs to hatchery unit. The capacity of hatchery should be only one fourth of the setter unit. The racks seen in the setter unit is larger than hatchery unit. Care should be taken while changing the eggs in upside down direction. If this is not done properly, embryo may be affected. And also water sprayer is used to maintain the humidity.

Single deck cabinet incubator

Similar size eggs are kept in this type of incubator. In this type all eggs are kept in the setter for 24 or 25 days and then it is transferred to the hatcher. As the hatching of poults take place once in a week only 3 setter and 1 hatcher is required (3:1 ratio). If hatching of poults takes place two times a week then 6setter and 1 hatcher is required (6:1 ratio). In this hygienic maintenance of incubator is very important.

Walk in incubator

In this type, the working person can go inside the incubator sets the eggs and can come back.

❑❑❑

Chapter 35

Sequence of Operations In A Hatchery

Collection of eggs from the farm
↓
Selection of eggs for hatching
↓
Cleaning of eggs (fumigation)
↓
Storage — Temperature 57-59^{0}F, Humidity 70-80% } 7 days
↓
↓
Removal of eggs from the storage room and allowing it to sweat and dry
Setter room
↓
↓ Temperature 99.5-100^{0}F & Humidity 70-75%
↓
Keeping the eggs in the rack of setter
↓
Fumigation of eggs in setter
↓

Candling of eggs (7th and 24th day)
↓
Transfer to hatchery (25th day)
Hatchery room
↓
↓ Temperature 99.5° F&
↓ Humidity 70-75%
Hatching of eggs (28th day)
↓
Removal of hatchery waste
↓
Poult sexing
↓
Vaccination
↓
Sale of turkey poults

Candling

Candling is done to determine the fertility of eggs; growth of embryo and also its quality. In a dark room, by means of electric bulb the quality of eggs is identified. This room should be well ventilated. The egg is kept at the distance of one foot from the eye and from the table. The light rays are made to pass through the eggs. The broader end is kept in upward direction and the egg should be turned fastly, so that the inner parts of eggs will move and embryo is checked.

In a dark room, wooden box with a hole in the shape of egg is used. The egg is placed in the hole and by means of 60 watt bulb the inner parts of egg is observed.

After the eggs are kept for incubation, candling should be done twice and infertile eggs should be removed. Similarly, on 5th or 7th day and on 24th day when the eggs are transferred to hatcher candling should be done.

Candling (day)	Changes in the embryo	Remarks
8th day	Eggs will be clear Red or black spot in the eggs Red ring in the eggs	No growth of embryo Early embryonic death Early embryonic death
After 8th day	Blood vessels are seen	Embryonated egg
10-16th day	Dark lines are noticed	Death of embryo
27-28th day	In the air cell, well developed beak of embryo is observed	Stage of chick hatching

Separation of Poults from the Hatchery and Sexing of Poult

Poults should be removed from the hatchery only when they are completely dried. If they are kept in the hatchery for prolonged period then there will be water loss and poults become weak. After removing the debris, the poults should be separated based on their quality. Poults with bright eyes, strong legs and well-developed feathers are separated as better quality. There should not be any congenital anomaly. After which sexing should be done.

Poult Sexing

In day old turkey poults sexing is done by Japanese heat sexing method. In this method male testicles are identified and sexing is done. But testis in day old turkey poults will not be developed completely. So it requires experience. Normally, sex identification is done between 12-14 weeks of age based on physical appearance.

Supply of Turkey Poults to the Farm

Turkey poults from the hatchery are supplied to the farms by means of poult boxes. In poult box, 12, 25, 50, or100 poults can be placed and supplied. Along with the poult box the guide for poult management and register should be sent.

□□□

Chapter 36

Location and Hatchery Design

For the effective functioning of hatchery, its location and construction is very important. Also the hygienic of hatchery is based on construction.

Location of Hatchery

The electricity, water, transport and labour facilities should be available in the site selected for hatchery. And also, the hatchery should be away from the other farms to avoid the spread of disease.

Office Room

The office room should be spacious and well ventilated. This room should be connected to the snure room where equipments, lead and registers are kept.

Working Place

This includes egg receiving room, egg assembly and traying hall, hatchery room, and chick sexing room and washing room. The process flow is a hatchery should be in a linear fashion from clean to dirty area.

Egg Storage Room

This room should be easily accessible to transport be so that the eggs can be received directly. This room should be large enough to store maximum number of eggs for 1 or 2 weeks. There should be many racks and the entire room should be air-conditioned.

Fumigation Room

Before keeping the eggs in the incubator, it should be fumigated. This is carried out to increase the hatchability. More number of eggs can be kept in this room. The entry of air should be restricted in the fumigation room. There should be extractor to remove the air inside the room.

Egg receiving and Incubator Room

Capacity of egg receiving room should be more, so that more number of eggs can be placed. All the elements should be kept in the right hand side for easier access to work. The tables in egg receiving room and egg assembly and traying hall should be in proper height so that work burden is reduced.

Incubator Room

There should be good access from incubator room to other rooms by means of sliding doors in the work side of the hatchery. This occupies lesser space and prevents the breakage of eggs. As far as possible reduce the use of glass windows and doors. The ceiling should be at the height of 15 feet. To ensure good ventilation throughout the incubator room, there should be at least 2 feet gap between the incubator frame and the wall. The distance between two rows of incubator should be 6 feet.

Setter size

Size of the setter is based on the following factors:

- Input cost
- Maintenance cost

- Space availability
- Spread of infection

Poult Sexing Room

The temperature of the room should be between 65 to 70°F. The rooms should be well ventilated and must have easily washable shelves to hold the poult boxes. Each table must be well equipped with high-powered overhead light that is adjustable for height. The sexing room must be provided with ample washing facilities.

Sales Room

This room must have direct access from the sexing room. The room should have a door leading directly to the road or hard standing pavement for vehicles. It should also be comfortable for the staff.

Other Rooms

There should be bathrooms and rest rooms for the workers.

Generator Shed

One or more standby source of electricity apart from the main supply source is requires for the hatchery. The room should be sufficiently large, well ventilated, and adjacent to the hatchery and with an easy access to the road. Sufficient space should be there inside the room to keep the reserve stock of fuel and necessary spare parts.

Washing Room

There should be facilities for cleaning the equipments. Cleaning of rubber slippers and dress wears can also be done.

Store Room

The room should be large enough and well planned for the racks to provide space for various hatchery items like poult boxes, packing materials, spare incubator fittings. Good lighting facilities and access to the road is also desirable.

Waste Room

This room should be away from other buildings. Cleaning of this room should be easy.

□□□

Chapter 37

Hatchery Hygiene

The hygienic maintenance of hatchery prevents the spread of the disease. Factors responsible for the spread of the disease are,

- Egg shell
- Endo and ectoparasites
- Cockroach
- Workers, their dresses and hand dirt

In the hatchery the disease spreads through the eggs, visitors, and vehicles. Before receiving the egg boxes in the hatchery, they should be Spraged with disinfectant. Before allowing the visitors inside the hatchery, they should clean their legs with disinfectant. Similarly vehicles should also be cleaned. The egg boxes that are sent from the hatchery should not be taken back. If it is a plastic box then it can be reused only after cleaning with disinfectant.

Building Maintenance

Should be kept clean.

Keep the floor and walls free from cobwebs and dirt.

Workers Hygiene

The workers should keep their clothes neat and clean. They should maintain separate clothes in hatchery. They should keep their hands, legs and head clean.

Hygienic Maintenance of Incubator and Fumigation of Eggs

The eggs racks in the incubator should be kept clean. And also, the hatchery equipment should be kept clean. The incubator should be cleaned with disinfectant once the poults are removed.

When To Do Fumigation?

- Before keeping the eggs in the storage room
- After keeping the eggs in the setter
- After changing the eggs from setter to hatcher, the setter should be fumigated
- After keeping the eggs in the hatcher
- After hatching of poults, the wastes in the hatchery should be removed and fumigated

Formaldehyde

To clean the instruments and to prevent the spread of disease, formaldehyde fumigation should be done. Method of generating the formaldehyde gas is,

- Potassium permanganate method
- Formalin sieve cloth method
- Para formaldehyde method
- Evaporation of formalin method

Potassium Permanganate Method

In this method, formalin and potassium permanganate are used. This will produce gas. Varying concentrations of potassium permanganate and formalin mixture is used for fumigation. They are,

Method 1

53ml of formalin (37.5%) and 35gm potassium permanganate is used for every 100 cubic feet of space.

Method 2

For every 100 cubic feet, 43ml of formalin (37.5%) and 21gm potassium permanganate mixture is used.

Method 3

For every 100 cubic feet, 45ml of formalin and 30gm potassium permanganate mixture is used.

Formalin Sieve Cloth Method

In this method, formalin and 36 feet sieve cloth is used. The sieve cloth is dipped in the formalin and it is hanged below the electric fan for 3 hours.

Para Formaldehyde Method

When the Para formaldehyde powder is placed in an electric pan with the thermostatic control at 150^0 F, formaldehyde gas is released. For every 100 cubic feet, 28 grams of formaldehyde is required.

Evaporation of Formalin Method

A 40% formalin solution is often used in regulated quantities for the fumigation of hatchers during the hatching period. Some hatchers are fitted with a special tray or cup for this purpose or the formalin may be placed in a container on the incubator floor.

Method of Fumigation

- The setter and the hatchery instruments should be kept in airtight room and fumigated. The electric fan should be present in the fumigation chamber. This helps in the spread of formaldehyde gas that is released from the formalin and potassium permanganate.
- Once the eggs are kept in the setter, the fumigation should be done only after 6 - 10 hours. Time taken for fumigation is 20 minutes.
- The formalin is poured in the vessel with potassium permanganate and kept in the room, which is to be fumigated.

- The vessels with formalin and potassium permanganate should be close to electric fan.
- Once the poults are removed from the hatchery, fumigation should be done within 30 minutes.

Time taken for fumigation

S.No	Fumigation of	Time required (minutes)
1	Hatching eggs	20
2	Eggs in the setter	20
3	Poults in the hatcher	3
4	Incubator room	30
5	Hatchery room	30
6	Poult box	30

Points To Be Noted During Fumigation

- The incubator room should be kept closed and no one should enter the room.
- While handling the formalin, rubber gloves should be used.
- They should wear masks

Removal of Debris from Setter and Hatcher

After removing the waste the setter & hatchery have to be cleaned with disinfectant.

Maintenance of Sexing Room

The person has involved in poult sexing should not enha other rooms. His clothes should be clean and should wear only rubber slippers. Table used for poult sexing must have metal tops so that they can be efficiently cleaned and disinfected as often necessary. The table should be cleaned with disinfectant between each batch of poults.

Prevention of Rodents, Insects, Cockroach and Bandicoots

Buildings

- The basement level should be at least 3 feet high from the ground level.
- There should not be any gap between floor and the wall.

- In windows, the gap between the two iron bars should not be more than ¼ feet. If the gap is more, then the window is to be netted.
- Any holes in the floors and walls should be closed.

Rodenticide

Warfarin, zinc can be used.

Ratrap

This can be used to reduce the rodent menanee.

Insecticides

The floor, ceilings and walls of the hatchery buildings should be sprayed with insecticides. Normally in well-managed hatchery buildings meets are not found.

❑❑❑

Chapter 38

Problems Encounted during Incubation and Its Control

The problems faced at the time of incubation are due to the improper management of hatchery, handling of eggs and improper management of breeding stock, including temperature, humidity, ventilation and turning of eggs in the incubator. The major problem associated with low hatchability is intractive eggs. They are due to age of turkey, proportion of male and female turkeys

Factors responsible for the death of the chicks at the time of incubation:

- Genetic makeup
- Management of incubator
- Hygiene
- Improper handling of eggs
- Nutritional deficiency

Mostly, the mortality of poults takes place when they come out of the shell. This is mainly due to the unhygienic maintenance of the hatchery.

Problems faced at the time of incubation

Problems	Reasons	Prevention
Infertile eggs	Improper proportion of male and female turkey used for mating	Optimum proportion of male and female turkey should be used
	Poor nutrition sup plied to the tom turkey	Proper nutrition should be supplied
	Competition between the tom turkeys at the time of mating	The turkeys used for breeding should be kept in separate rooms
	Damage to the comb and wattle of the turkey	Proper space requirement s hould be supplied to the breeding stock
	Using old tom turkey	The young turkeys to replace the old turkeys. Sterile males should be removed. (Spiking)
	Storage of eggs for long time. Improper temperature, humidity and ventilation in the storage rooms	The hatching eggs should not be stored for more than 7 days.
	High or low temperature in the incubator	Thermometer and temperature control system is used to regulate the temperature
	Improper fumigation	The chemicals should be used in proper concentration. Eggs m ust never be fumigated between 24 th and 96th hour after setting
Death of embryo inside the egg shell	High or low temperature in the incubator	Thermometer and temperature control system is used to regulate the temperature. Power supply should be maintained
	Turning of eggs when not done in the incubator	Turning should be done 3 or 5 times per day. Turning should not be done in same direction.
	Improper nutritional supplement to the breeding	Proper nutrition should be supplied to the breeding stock.

	stock. This leads to the death of embryo within 10 to 14 days of incubation	
	Improper ventilation in the incubator	Proper ventilation should be provided.
	Pullorum and other diseases	The eggs of disease resistant turkeys should be used for hatching
Not hatched but broken eggs	Not enough humidity in the incubator	Increase the vapourization of water in the water plates or sprinkle water over the eggs
	Humidity is at the higher level	Wet bulb thermometer is used to check the humidity
	Nutrition deficient problems	Proper nutrition should be supplied
Early hatching	Temperature of the incubator is at the higher level	Thermometer and temperature control system is used to regulate the temperature. Regular power supply should be maintained.
Late hatching	Lower level of temperature in the incubator	
Sticky turkey poults	Lower level of temperature in the incubator	Maintain the temperature even when there is no power supply
Poults with congenital anomaly	Temperature of the incubator is at the higher level	Thermometer and temperature control system is used to regulate the temperature
	Lower level of temperature in the incubator	Maintain the temperature even when there is no power supply
	Turning of eggs is not done in the incubator	Turning should be done 3 or 5 times per day. Turning should not be done in same direction.
Weak turkey poults	Temperature of the incubator is at the higher level	Thermometer and temperature control system is used to regulate the temperature. Regular power supply should be maintained.
Poults with higher respiratory rate	Temperature of the incubator is at the higher level	

Mortality of poults	Smaller sized eggs are kept for incubation	Only medium sized eggs should be used for hatching
	Lower level of humidity in the incubator	Increase the vapourization of water in the water plates or sprinkle water over the eggs
	More amount of chemicals used for fumigation	The chemicals should be used in proper concentration. Eggs must never fumigated between 24th and 96th hour after setting
	Higher level of humidity in the incubator	Conversion of water to vapourizer should be reduced
	Spread of disease	Turkey poults should be checked and diseased poults should be treated or removed
	Lower level of temperature in the incubator	Thermometer and temperature control system is used to regulate the temperature. Regular power supply should be maintained.
	Improper ventilation in the incubator	Proper ventilation should be provided
All eggs kept in the incubator do not hatch on the same day	The eggs kept for hatching are of different ages	Do not store the eggs for more than 10 days

To avoid the problems in the breeder turkey farms, the egg production in the farm, the disease incidence, mortality percentage, and weight of the egg, quality of eggshell, hatching ability, feed intake and immunity level should be recorded in the registers regularly. And also candling should be done within a week and infertile eggs should be removed. The nutritional deficiency should be avoided in the breeder stock.

□□□

Chapter 39

Economics for Breeder Turkey and Hatchery (50 Females and 10 Males)

Assumptions

Cost of one breeder turkey

1. If cost of one kg live turkey for breeding is Rs.100, then the cost of tom, which weighs 4.5kg and hen, which weighs 3.5kg, are Rs.450 and Rs.350 respectively. Total number turkeys required for breeding are 50 females and 10 males. They are perclosed at Point of Lay.
2. Age of first egg is 24 weeks. Hatchy eggs are collected during the 30-52 weeks.
3. Number of eggs obtained from a hen turkey is 100.
4. Number of poults obtained from a female is 70.
5. Amount of feed consumed by the female at the time of egg laying for one week is 1.05kg. Then for 28 weeks it is about 30kg.
6. Amount of feed consumed by Tom for one week is 1.4kg, so total amount of feed consumed is 39kg for 28 weeks.
7. Rate of one kg feed is Rs.18.

1. Fixed cost

a. Building construction cost: The space requirement for one turkey is 5sq.ft then for 60turkeys it is 300sq.ft. Cost for one sq.ft is Rs.75. (Thatched roof shed) then cost for 300sq.ft is Rs. 22,500.00

b. Space required for hatchery is 200sq.ft. Cost of construction for one sq.ft is

Rs.1000 then for 200sq.ft it is Rs. 2,00,000.00

c. Equipment cost: setter cum and hatcher

Capacity of setter are 800 eggs and hatcher are200 eggs

Rs. 60,000.00

d. Cost of feeder and waterer for one turkey is Rs.15 and then for 60 turkeys Rs. 900.00

Total (A) Rs. 2,83,400.00

2. Variable cost

a. Cost of 50 breeding female and 10 male turkeys are

Rs. 22,000.00

b. Cost of feed: Feed requirement for 50 female are 1500kg and for 10 male are 390kg. Then total cost of the feed is

Rs. 34,020.00

c. Electricity cost Rs. 6,000.00

d. Medicine and vaccination cost for one turkey is Rs.10 then for 60 turkeys Rs. 600.00

e. Miscellaneous cost Rs. 1000.00

Total (B) Rs. 63,020.00

3. Returns

Number of poults obtained from one female turkey is 70 and then from 50 female are 3500 chicks. Rate one turkey poult is Rs.70 then for 3500 poults (C) Rs. 2,45,000.00

4. Income

Returns – variable cost (C –B) Rs. 1,81,980.00

□□□

Chapter 40

Hatching Ability of Turkey Eggs

Poult hatching ability can be identified by the following formula:

$$\text{Fertility}(\%) = \frac{\text{Total number of fertile eggs}}{\text{Total number of eggs produced or set for incubation}} \times 100$$

The poults hatching percentage is defined as a total number of poults produced to the total number of fertile eggs.

$$\text{Hatchability}(\%) = \frac{\text{Total number of poults hatched}}{\text{Total number of fertile eggs set}} \times 100$$

By the following tabular column, eggs produced by hen turkey, fertility and hatching ability of the poults can be identified.

Egg production

Egg laying period	Number of eggs produced from a turkey for a week	Total number of eggs produced from a turkey during its entire egg laying period
1	2.80	2.80
2	4.95	7.75
3	5.32	13.07
4	5.15	18.22
5	5.14	23.36
6	5.18	28.54
7	5.18	33.72
8	5.16	38.88
9	5.13	44.01
10	5.08	49.09
11	5.00	54.09
12	4.92	59.01
13	4.83	63.84
14	4.74	68.58
15	4.63	73.21
16	4.54	77.75
17	4.45	82.20
18	4.37	86.57
19	4.28	90.85
20	4.19	95.04
21	4.10	99.14
22	4.00	103.14
23	3.90	107.04
24	3.80	110.84
25	3.70	114.54
26	3.60	118.14

True fertility %	% of eggs hatched from fertile egg	% of eggs hatched from total eggs kept for incubation
92.0	85.0	74.6
94.2	87.7	79
94.2	89.9	82.5
95.8	91.4	84.3
96.1	92.1	85.1
96.2	92.3	85.5
96.3	92.1	85.4
96.3	91.9	85.1
96.2	91.7	84.8
96.1	91.4	84.4
95.9	91.1	84.0
95.8	90.7	83.5
95.7	90.2	83
95.6	89.7	82.3
95.4	89.2	81.6
95.2	88.6	80.8
95.0	88.1	80.1
94.7	87.6	79.2
94.4	87	78.4
94.4	86.5	77.6
93.7	86.1	76.8
93.5	85.6	76.1
93.1	85.1	75.3
92.7	84.6	74.4
92.3	83.5	73
91.9	82.7	71.9

Hatching ability		
Number of poults obtained from a female turkey for a week %	**Total number of poults obtained from a female turkey during its entire production period %**	**Age in weeks**
2.09	2.09	33
3.91	6.00	34
4.39	10.39	35
4.34	14.73	36
4.37	19.10	37
4.43	23.53	38
4.42	27.96	39
4.39	32.35	40
4.35	36.70	41
4.29	40.99	42
4.20	45.19	43
4.11	49.29	44
4.01	53.30	45
3.90	57.20	46
3.78	60.98	47
3.67	64.65	48
3.56	68.21	49
3.46	71.68	50
3.36	75.03	51
3.25	78.28	52
3.15	81.43	53
3.04	84.48	54
2.94	87.41	55
2.83	90.24	56
2.70	92.94	57
2.59	95.53	58

REGISTERS FOR HATCHING ABILITY

S.No	Remarks	Date of incubation	Date of hatching	Early embryonic mortality No.	Early embryonic mortality %	Late embryonic mortality No.	Late embryonic mortality %	No. of Weak turkey poults	No. of Good turkey poults	Total No. of poults	Hatching ability % Total eggs for incubation	Hatching ability % Fertile eggs

Egg maintenance register

Date	Opening balance	Received eggs	Total No. Eggs	No. Kept for incubation	No. of Table eggs	No. of unwanted eggs (small and large sized eggs)	No. of broken eggs	Total wastage	Closing Balance	Remarks

About the Authors

Dr. D. Thyagarajan being specialised in poultry science with doctorate degree, having more than 80 research articles, 130 research paper presentations, 126 popular articles, 26 books edited, authored 10 books, generated six technologies, completed nine research projects as Principal Investigator and recognised nationally with ICAR "Outstanding extension scientist/worker award" for the year 1996-1998. Right now, the author holding two assignments as Dean, Faculty of Food Sciences and Director of Research, Tamil Nadu Veterinary and Animal Sciences University. Completed 32 years of University service from Assistant Professsor to present position. Currently involved in many positions for policy development of state and centre.

The author has completed ICAR funded scheme " Evolving optimum management practices and nutritional requirement of turkey" which outlined 42 biological experiments. He has established , " Package of practice for scientific turkey farming". He was responsible for technology dissemination to turkey farmers in Kancheepuram district. He was instrumental to create microentrepreneur avenues in scientific turkey farming among the resource poor women. He has completed DBT funded project, " Poverty alleviation through scientific turkey farming in selected rural areas of Kancheepuram District of Tamil Nadu ". He has carried out lot of pioneer works in the turkey, and guinea fowl farming. His rich experience and scientific knowledge gathered over the years is outlined in the present book in different segments as scientific turkey management, turkeys feed and feeding and hatchery management. He has carried out lot of pioneer works in the turkey, and guinea fowl farming.

Dr. A. Ashok is a Assistant Professor of Poultry Science of Tamil Nadu Veterinary and Animal Sciences University, Chennai. He has over 13 years of experience in teaching, research and extension activities. He is a recipient of senior fellowship in poultry science awarded by ICAR. He is also recipient of Ms.Venkatehwara Hatcheries gold medal for the first rank in M.V.Sc. Poultry science in College of Veterinary Science, Hyderabad, APAU.He was also awarded the Ms.Venkatehwara Hatcheries gold medal for the best Ph.D. thesis in the field by TANUVAS. He has published several technical papers/articles to his credit. He has also authored/edited over 10 books. He is a life member of several professional societies.

